EARLY PRAISE FOR SANDRO GALEA'S *WELL*

"Galea elevates our understanding of what forces influence our health and shape our well-being, writing with sensitivity, nuance and authority."
—Joseph Amon, Drexel University, former director of Health and Human Rights Division, Human Rights Watch

"Conversations around healthcare mean more if we live in a society that actively values health—not just medicine. Sandro Galea's case for change in America is bold, disarming, and eminently achievable. Well is the starting point for a conversation we need to have."
—Jeff Arnold, Chairman and CEO, Sharecare

"*Well* should be required reading for anyone interested in understanding what is necessary for health in the U.S. Galea applies his remarkable breadth of knowledge to some of the most complex issues facing humanity—and does so with such clarity and insight that even the most complex topics suddenly seem crystal clear."
—John Auerbach, President and CEO, Trust for America's Health

"Galea moves beyond a numbing rhetoric of numbers to tell how societal forces mold people's health."
—Mary Bassett, Harvard University, former New York City Health Commissioner

"A brilliant exposé of the societal factors that profoundly impact individual and population health."
—Georges C. Benjamin, Executive Director, American Public Health Association

"A radical new perspective on the true drivers of health—and a set of truly disruptive conclusions to inspire those designing health systems. A defining manifesto for the years ahead."
—Arnaud Bernaert, World Economic Forum

"A sensitive and nuanced perspective on often overlooked issues—compassion, fairness, freedom—that matter most to our health."
—David Blumenthal, President, The Commonwealth Fund

"For 45 years I have fought for equity, compassion, and inclusion in mental health, so I am thrilled to see Sandro Galea's *Well* take the revolutionary and compelling stance that these principles can have a more beneficial effect upon public health than any scientific discovery."
— Rosalynn Carter, former First Lady

"Explains, convincingly, that history is the principal determinant of population health and why collective action to promote socio-economic justice is the most effective way to improve it."

—Daniel M. Fox, President Emeritus, Milbank Memorial Fund

"A fresh, rich, and practical discussion of health as a social imperative and the multiple forces that shape it. From one of the most creative and influential thinkers in the public health field, this book will become an essential companion to practitioners and scholars alike."

—Julio Frenk, President, University of Miami

"Sandro Galea's work deftly captures the disconnect between healthcare spending and what actually determines our health. His work is a clarion call for changes in how we invest to make America healthier."

—Paul S. Grogan, President and CEO, The Boston Foundation

"With healthcare increasingly a political football, *Well* guides us toward what is truly needed for a healthier world. Its power comes from Galea's remarkable ability to draw on the power of individual stories and lived experience to humanize the issues and inspire commitment to improved health for all."

—Margaret Hamburg, former FDA Commissioner

"*Well* is the essence of good health for all and a call to action to get us there. A must-read for all those who share this universal goal."

—Ruth J. Katz, The Aspen Institute

"Vested in both personal experience and stark data, Galea's *Well* provides a refreshingly accessible, novel and important break down of many of the reasons why we really get sick—and the opportunities to be well."

—Vanessa Kerry, Seed Global Health

"A clear and compelling case that health inequities resulting from environmental, societal, and political forces are holding all of us back. It's time to reinvest in our health—not just our healthcare."

— Gina McCarthy, Harvard University, former EPA Administrator

"Weaving together history, philosophy, social science data, and current events, Galea has created a powerful narrative advocating for a more holistic understanding of population health."

—Travis McCready, President and CEO,
Massachusetts Life Sciences Center

"An engagingly written and heartfelt cry for us all to recognize the connection between our collection action and personal health."

—David Miller, C40 Cities Climate Leadership Group,
former Mayor of Toronto

WELL

WELL

WHAT WE NEED TO TALK ABOUT WHEN WE TALK ABOUT HEALTH

SANDRO GALEA

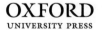

OXFORD
UNIVERSITY PRESS

OXFORD

UNIVERSITY PRESS

Oxford University Press is a department of the University of Oxford. It furthers
the University's objective of excellence in research, scholarship, and education
by publishing worldwide. Oxford is a registered trade mark of Oxford University
Press in the UK and certain other countries.

Published in the United States of America by Oxford University Press
198 Madison Avenue, New York, NY 10016, United States of America.

Library of Congress Cataloging-in-Publication Data
Names: Galea, Sandro, author.
Title: Well : what we need to talk about when we talk about health / Sandro Galea.
Description: Oxford ; New York : Oxford University Press, [2019] |
Includes bibliographical references and index.
Identifiers: LCCN 2018043016 | ISBN 9780190916831 (hardback)
Subjects: LCSH: Public health—United States. | Medical care—United States. |
BISAC: SELF-HELP / General. | MEDICAL / Alternative Medicine. |
MEDICAL / Public Health.
Classification: LCC RA445 .G35 2019 | DDC 362.10973—dc23
LC record available at https://lccn.loc.gov/2018043016

1 3 5 7 9 8 6 4 2

Printed by Sheridan Books, Inc., United States of America

This book is dedicated, as always, to Isabel Tess Galea, Oliver Luke Galea, and Dr. Margaret Kruk.

CONTENTS

I am a physician and an epidemiologist (a doctor who studies how diseases spread) by profession. I am also an immigrant, twice over, and a father.

I was born in Malta, a small island about one-tenth the size of Rhode Island, located in the Mediterranean between Sicily and Tunisia. During my childhood, Malta went through a period of political unrest, mass civil disobedience, and violence. The changes did not bode well for my family, and we left the island in 1985, when I was a teenager.

We moved to Canada, which at the time was one of two countries (Australia was the other) accepting Maltese immigrants. There we lived with my aunt, who had immigrated previously, in a Toronto suburb called Scarborough, where a fair number of immigrants lived (and still do). Later we moved to a housing project nearby. I did a year and a bit of high school, then attended Scarborough College, a commuter campus of the University of Toronto.

I went to medical school in Canada and then practiced medicine in a rural part of Northern Canada. I also worked in places like Papua New Guinea and the Philippines and with Doctors Without Borders in Somalia. When I was approaching 30, I immigrated to the United States to study public health. I have since made my professional living here, conducting research and teaching at the University of Michigan, Columbia University, and now Boston University.

My children are fully American, and I am now very much at home here. But I have little doubt that my sensibility is shaped by a personal journey that gives me deep empathy with vulnerable and marginalized groups. At the same time, my journey imbues me with genuine optimism about the potential to always improve the human condition. And, by professional orientation, I want us to be better on health. Experience living around the world has taught me that health is universally valued and that all members of the human family wish to be healthier. My training in medicine and public health tells me that we can do just that, provided we first change what we talk about when we talk about health. That is what this book is about.

—Sandro Galea
July 18, 2018
Boston

In 1977, NASA launched the unmanned Voyager One space probe, the goal of which was to explore the outermost reaches of space and transmit data back to earth.[1] On board was a gold-plated record containing a range of sounds that would convey, to any alien being that discovered it, the breadth and diversity of the human experience on earth.[2] One song on the record is "Dark Was the Night, Cold Was the Ground," a recording from 1927 by the blues singer Blind Willie Johnson.

Blind Willie Johnson had a difficult life.[3,4] The story goes that when Willie was seven years old, as his father was beating Willie's stepmother over allegations of infidelity, the step-mother angrily threw lye in Willie's face, blinding him. Willie experienced poverty throughout the life that followed, getting by on money earned playing music and preaching in the streets. In 1945, his house burned to the ground.[5] With nowhere to go, he lived in the ruins, sleeping on a damp bed. Amid these living conditions he soon caught malaria and died. His wife said that he had been refused treatment at a hospital, either because he was blind or because he was black.[6]

When I tell this story to groups, I ask them a question: what killed Blind Willie Johnson? The answer may seem obvious: malaria killed Blind Willie Johnson. If he had received treatment for it, Blind Willie would have lived.

But would he have lived much longer? Anyone who appreciates the sum of hardships that were building up in Blind Willie's life will recognize that if malaria had not killed him on September 18, 1945, something else was likely going to kill him soon thereafter. In fact, one might fairly argue that he was killed by poverty, by racism, by domestic violence, by homelessness, and by limited access to care. And, in this regard, he was not alone. Today, black children in America are far more likely to witness domestic violence than white ones, and while doctors may not be able to turn patients away on account of race anymore, pernicious gaps in treatment remain.

Blind Willie Johnson's health was shaped by being born at a certain time, in a certain place, in a certain skin, under certain social and economic circumstances. The sum of all these factors is what ultimately defined his life experience and killed him at an early age.

On hearing this story, most will regret what happened to Johnson, lamenting how such things continue to happen to people today. One may even hope to do something to help those who are affected by adverse conditions today so that those people can be healthier.

These are admirable sentiments, but they miss a core truth: we are all Blind Willie Johnson. Each of us is shaped by the conditions around us—the combination of place, time, power, money, and connections, by what we know, and by the compassion of the people we encounter. And, importantly, our health depends on these things, too.

This book aims to make this case: that our health is not defined by things like seeing doctors or taking medicines or getting in our 5,000 steps a day. Rather, it's defined by the full spectrum of our life circumstances, from the families we come from to the neighborhoods where we live to the people we see and the choices we make. And unless we understand those forces, our health is never going to improve.

The room for improvement in Americans' health is well documented. In fact, by most measures, American health is worse than that of any other rich country. Child mortality in the United States is about 7 per 1,000; in Finland it's 2 per 1,000. A child born today in America can expect to live until age 79; in Japan, that child would live to 84. Yet, somehow, we spend nearly twice as much as Japan does on health per capita.[7]

Most well-informed Americans are aware of this trend. It has become accepted that we live sicker and die earlier than people in other rich countries. What most do not realize is that this is a relatively new development. While the United States has made continuing progress on improving life expectancy and reducing mortality from various diseases, these improvements have occurred at a much slower rate than in other countries over the past 40 years. For example, Chilean life expectancy was 68 in 1980; it was 81 by 2014. By comparison, U.S. life expectancy was 74 in 1980, and, by 2014, it lagged behind Chile's at 79. And the United States is not just faring worse than other high-income countries. In 1980, Cuban life expectancy was 74. In 2005, it was 79, higher than 77 in the United States.[7] Today, children born in America are likelier to live shorter lives than children born in a range of other countries, including Singapore (life expectancy 83) and Greece (life expectancy 81).[8]

Is this because Americans care less about health than do people in other countries? Far from it. The United States spent $3.3 trillion in 2016 on health.[9] That is the same as the entire gross domestic product of Germany.[10] America spends about 18% of its annual gross domestic product on health. The country that spends the second most is Switzerland, which spends 12%. Most of the 37 countries that are part of the Organization for Economic Cooperation and Development spend somewhere around 9%.[11]

Much of Americans' health expenditures go toward doctors and medicines—that is, money spent on getting better after we are sick. The inefficiency of this approach shines a light on how Americans historically conflate the concept of health with the practice of medicine and how our national health conversation is dominated by a belief that treating illness is somehow easier or better than preventing that illness in the first place.

It is hard to think of any other aspect of American life where the country's shortcomings are as stark as with its health, let alone one where it would be remotely as accepted. Would Americans accept spending more than anyone else on its military if it was understood that our military was weaker than those of other countries? How would we feel if we continued to spend more on our military over a period of decades only to fall further and further behind other countries? It would probably amount to a national crisis and prompt some real soul-searching and hand-wringing around why we have been spending ever more while getting ever less.

All this happens because we think about health in the wrong way. We think that improving health is an individual enterprise focused on the individual. We think that lifestyle will amount to living longer as long as we can afford all the medicines we need to keep going. But study after study shows that our country's health output per dollar is worse than any of our peer countries, and study after study also shows that efforts to change our lifestyle generally fall short just a few months after we make these efforts. This means we've been spending our money on ineffectual, finger-wagging efforts to modify behaviors, then later on medicine to help us after we get sick. Based on the evidence, that appears to be the wrong approach.

This book is about the forces around us that shape health, most of which we do not think about. These are forces that are typically not in the health discussion—but, based on research, should be. To take that statement a step further, this book is about factors that have to align with the goal of creating the healthiest possible people if we are to reap the benefits of our investment in health.

We spend an inordinate amount of money on health, yes. Most of the time we have been spending that money incorrectly. We have been spending on trying to do things by ourselves, to change behaviors that aren't likely to change in light of the vortex of factors that contributed to the behaviors in the first place. We have been spending our money on medicine, looking to cure ourselves after we have become sick, rather than investing in the things that will prevent us from getting sick in the first place.

The fact that we spend so much and get so relatively little for it is evidence that we cannot buy our way out of this problem. Despite having the best hospitals in the world, Americans will still get sick more than people living in other countries and will then die at a younger age. And, for all our best intentions in health—to eat better, to exercise more—we will keep falling short because our world and environment are not aligned to encourage us to do these things. The society we have created is simply not oriented to keep us healthy.

Until our world is oriented in a way that is conducive to health, we will continue to fall behind on health and never come close to realizing our full potential, even amid extraordinary health-related spending. Our efforts to make ourselves healthy without a world around us that encourages health will never be sufficient. At the end of the day, it does not matter so much how great our hospitals are or how advanced our technology. Our health is determined by, and limited by, the world in which we live.

The good news is that introducing the matters of actual consequence to our dialogues around health doesn't cost any more than we're already spending. But it will require that we pay greater attention to certain things than we do now, and that sort of behavior change is no small trick. The goal here has to be to shift what we talk about when we talk about health. The chapters of this book show how what we value, how we live, where we live, and who is in power are all drivers of our health, individually and collectively. It explains how, until we have a more just world, health will continue to suffer. And it explains why forces as abstract as empathy and humility matter for our health—and, critically, why we must embrace their influence.

My bias—as a writer, as a doctor, as an immigrant, as an academic, as a father—is that I hope to live in a healthier world, for all. In this book, I attempt to explain the various factors in our broader context that we know create good health. It's important to note that I am not interested in disease, and I seldom talk about sickness. I am interested in health, in the creation of a world where as many of us as possible are healthy for as long as possible.

While our health is personal, I am interested in how everyone, as many people as possible, can be as healthy as possible for as long as possible. To that end, I hope that this book can serve as a meditation of sorts, guiding the reader to better understand the forces that actually shape our health. From there, maybe we can turn to investing in these very forces and creating a healthier world.

In many ways, this book is a reflection of my own personal journey in health. I was born in Malta and immigrated to Canada, where I was trained as a physician in primary care medicine. I spent time working in rural and remote parts of the world, including Somalia, where I worked as a field physician with Doctors Without Borders. It was in Somalia in the late 1990s where I was truly immersed in the most acute form of clinical medicine: dealing with sick people coming through the door whose lives, literally, depended on me and what I did to help them. People whose malaria (and there was a lot of malaria) depended on my treating it properly in order for them to live.

While in Somalia, treating mostly preventable diseases and injuries, I felt very much like the proverbial man at the side of the river who sees one person drowning and jumps in to save her, then sees another person drowning and jumps in to save him, and then yet another person and jumps in to save her. After a while I stopped to ask: Who is throwing people in the river to begin with?

With that question began my academic journey. My professional life has been focused on finding out who is throwing people in the river and what I can do about that upstream influence so that we are not all drowning and depending on doctors to fish us out.

The forces around us are what throws us in the river. They are our past, money, power, place, people, love and hate, compassion, the choices we make, luck, fairness and justice, and our values. My hope is that if we all understand these forces a little bit better, we will have fewer people drowning in the river and that the Blind Willie Johnsons of the world will live another day.

ONE

THE PAST

*S*ofia was born to a mother who could not quite afford her. Financially insecure all her life, she gave birth at 17 and supported Sofia by working two jobs—one at a fast food restaurant, the other at a laundromat at the other end of the city. Because of her mother's long commute, and longer hours, Sofia's care fell largely to a cousin who allowed her to spend most of her time eating potato chips and watching television. Despite this indulgence, which left her slightly overweight, Sofia was by no means lazy. She always made sure the family apartment was clean and well-ordered, keeping everything neat while her mother was away. Yet there were limits to what she could do to ensure the cleanliness of her surroundings. Her home was close to the local bus depot, where, all day long, the vehicles pumped thick diesel fumes into the air. As a consequence, Sofia was plagued by severe asthma that often kept her from school. Her grades tended to be low, with the exception of math. When it came to numbers, she quickly surpassed her peers and even some of the students in the year ahead of her. Recognizing Sofia's potential, one of her teachers recommended her for special enrichment classes. Unfortunately, this meant someone would have to regularly drive Sofia home after school, and she had no such someone in her life. She never took the classes.

When she was about 16, Sofia became pregnant and dropped out of school. Her mother, still working two jobs, had not been around to counsel her about reproductive safety, and the cursory sexual education provided by Sofia's school emphasized abstinence far more than it did condoms. So, Sofia, still living under her mother's roof, followed in her mother's footsteps, working multiple low-wage jobs to make ends meet and support her daughter. The stress of these jobs and the pressures of young motherhood took a toll on her health. By the time she was 28, she was 40 pounds overweight, her asthma was worse, and she was diagnosed with type 2 diabetes. To cope with these conditions, she was soon prescribed three medications by her doctor. This strained her income and her capacity to help her mother keep up payments on the apartment. As time passed, and once her daughter became a bit more independent, Sofia was able to consolidate her work life into a single, stable job. She became the manager of a crew at a catering company. She enjoyed working with her team, earned good money, and often received praise from the company's owner. But the pace and physical nature of the work did no favors for her health. By her mid-40s, Sofia's asthma and diabetes were poorly controlled. She developed osteoarthritis in both knees—brought on by her extra weight. Her doctor told her she would soon need surgery to address these problems, which would take her off her feet and away from the work for which she had shown such aptitude. She tried to defer the surgery, and her doctor prescribed opioids for her knee pain. Sofia quickly developed a dependence on the drugs. After a fall at work, her doctor *told her that a corrective procedure could no longer wait. Sofia, at age 45, was now receiving regular medical attention and headed to early surgery.*

Sofia's story captures the essence of how our health is shaped by our past and how our past is, in turn, shaped by a range of social, economic, and environmental conditions. If we were to meet Sofia as our story leaves her—age 45, overweight, suffering from the combined effects of asthma, diabetes, and osteoarthritis—it would be easy to see how her physical challenges undermine her present health. It would be less easy to see how the circumstances of her personal history laid the groundwork for these challenges to emerge.

Sofia's medical picture at 45 is as much the result of her health in the years preceding as the day her surgery was deemed necessary. Her health is a product of her life, and her life, like all lives, is complex. Nutrition, culture, income, race, family dynamics, and educational attainment—all these factors are unique to individuals, and together they define our individual complexities. It should come as little surprise, then, that Sofia does not need surgery at age 45 because of any one issue; she needs it because of an accumulation of experiences that amount to her personal history up to this moment in time. What the Sofia story should make clear is that, while it may be tempting to ascribe her health issues to poor choices on her part, a more nuanced understanding of her personal history proves that any such interpretation is vastly simplistic and incomplete.

History teaches us that many of the conditions that shape our health are outside our control. There is little Sofia could have done, for example, to avoid asthma, with her home so close to dangerous pollutants. There is also little she could have done to educate herself about safe sex in the absence of any resources that would have helped her do so. And there is nothing she could have done to have been born into wealth and all the health advantages money can bring. Perhaps the most tragic aspect of Sofia's history is that it represents a cycle that her daughter is likely to repeat, just as Sofia's story came to mirror that of her own mother. In the United States, we like to tell ourselves that anyone can transcend the circumstances of his or her birth through the application of hard work. The data tell a different story. More than 40% of Americans who grew up at the bottom of the economic ladder remain there as adults, with only 4% managing to rise to the top.[1] Given this reality, Sofia's past will likely shape her daughter's future, just as her mother's past shaped hers.

Our health is also intergenerational, influenced by our parents' health and their parents' health. This influence starts to mold our health before we are even born, starting with how our parents' health determines our own experiences in utero. Low birth weight (LBW) is an example of this.[2] The term LBW is applied when a child is born weighing under 5 pounds, 8 ounces. A baby's chances of being born with LBW are closely linked with her mother's experiences during pregnancy. Parental substance use can contribute to LBW risk. So can age: giving birth under the age of 17 or above the age of 35 increases the likelihood of the child being born

with LBW. LBW is linked to low income, lack of education, and unemployment. It is also tied to stress, including
racialized stress—a 2017 study found that infants born to
Latina mothers in Iowa after the major immigration raid in
Postville had a 24% greater risk of LBW.[3,4] The potential
health effects of LBW are significant. The condition can lead
to a number of problems for the child later on, including obesity, diabetes, and heart disease. The influence of our past may
also run deeper than we suppose. Evidence suggests that even
the conditions of parents' early lives may affect their children's
health. Research has shown how, when children are exposed to
difficult socioeconomic conditions, it increases the risk that
their own children will develop asthma.[5]

Once we are born, the influence of our parents combines
with our own early experiences to set the stage for health
throughout our individual lives. Childhood trauma, for example, has been linked with significantly higher odds of later
marijuana and cocaine use.[6] Individuals who start drinking before the age of 14 are at greater lifetime risk for alcohol dependence.[7] But it is education that has perhaps the greatest effect on
our health trajectory through the years. In 2006, a 25-year-old
man without a high school diploma could expect to live more
than 9 years less than a 25-year-old man with a bachelor's degree or higher; this life expectancy gap was more than 8 years
for women.[8] The health risks of low education have even been
compared, in terms of their mortality, to the dangers posed by
smoking.[9]

This probably isn't news to anyone reading this. In fact, much of what's contained in this book is, perhaps, science that is familiar to educated readers. And yet, for all we know, we often cannot help but think that it is all inevitable, that it does not apply to us, or that with enough medicine we can buy our way out of our past and our circumstances and be as healthy as we want to be. But, in fact, we have no choice *but* to think about the past when we consider health.

When we ignore the past, we risk overlooking how the forces that shape our lives and our world also shape health across generations. It makes us less likely to address these conditions, feeding the sense (and the myth) that health is solely a product of our individual choices and the medicines we take. It has implications for where we invest and how we act.

Consider the U.S. National Institutes of Health (NIH), the U.S. government's highly funded agency for medical research. The NIH is made up of 27 institutes and centers, each tasked with studying a particular disease or physiological system, funded according to the burden and urgency of the specific diseases they address.[10] These organizations include a National Cancer Institute, a National Eye Institute, a National Institute of Mental Health, and a National Heart, Lung, and Blood Institute. All do important work. However, their scope is limited to the present. There are no institutes devoted to studying the cumulative influence of the past on health. In other words, the NIH is interested in Sofia's diabetes, but it has yet to fully reckon with the history that produced it, nor with the socioeconomic conditions that characterized this history. This orientation is to be expected for the NIH—it is a reasonable reflection of how we view health in our society. Disease, in the popular conception, has an immediacy to it. It seems to strike suddenly, like a storm. But the reality, of course, is that storms develop slowly over time, relying on the right set of weather conditions to give them the force to make landfall. Disease, too, requires conditions plus time to produce its effects. More often than not, we devote our attention to addressing these effects at the expense of addressing the time and conditions that created them. This approach distorts our view of disease, even leading us to blame sick people for their own poor health. We look at someone like Sofia and judge her present health without taking into account her past. We see her obesity and assume that she eats too much because she is weak-willed. We see her wheeze and dismiss her as a smoker too headstrong to care about the risks. We see her work a low-wage job and conclude that she is too unintelligent to do anything else.

These judgments are manifestly cruel. They are also common—common enough to serve as the basis for much of our public policy. They show why, if we do not think about the past when we think about health, it's not just Sofia's health that will not improve; it's our collective health.

The United States has a system of six federal programs that are designed to promote health among individuals and families of lesser means; these programs provide nutrition assistance, insurance coverage, and income subsidies, and are often housed under the umbrella term "welfare." In practice, the beneficiaries of welfare programs are doggedly antagonized and even penalized for their need, forced to repeatedly prove that their difficulties are not the products of their own low character. Our welfare policies are written and updated in ways that appear to assume laziness among those who would dare to use them: we implement Medicaid work requirements and drug tests and are skeptical of universal healthcare, with some decrying it as a socialist plot to make responsible healthy people subsidize the dissolute sick. This all represents an ahistorical view of health. It ignores generations of history—not just the history of individuals, but the history of a country where a deeply unequal past has given way to an only marginally less unequal present. Worse, these actions channel political will in the wrong direction, away from improving the conditions that truly shape health. When a politician criticizes someone like Sofia, he or she ignores the fact that the zoning policies of Sofia's city allowed a bus depot to be built next to her apartment building, causing her asthma. We don't ask critical questions, like why Sofia's mother could not elevate her family into the middle class despite working so hard she barely had time to see her child. We aren't troubled by the thought that we may be collectively responsible for this history, and this is evident in our inaction around the conditions that make it repeat itself. And as a result, we are less likely to see how ignoring history is a global problem, predicting and perpetuating cycles of violence and poverty that undermine the health of millions.

Failing to recognize the role of the past affects the health of all of us, even those fortunate enough to live unaffected by the factors that colored Sofia's life. Because if our federal funding focuses only on our medical needs *today*, as if they are lightning strikes, then we'll never understand how the car accident we happened to be involved in when we were children can increase our risk of diabetes and depression in adulthood—and, most important, how we can prevent these conditions after these experiences. And if we focus only on diet plans that aim to improve our weight today, we will not devote any attention to making sure we are not exposed to the calorie-dense, nutrient-poor foods as children that will saddle us with obesity throughout our life.

To avoid this thinking, we must address the structures that surround us every day—the conditions that shape who we are and who we will become. A closer look at racism in America, for example, reminds us how history (in this case, slavery) can become embedded in the systems that organize our society and in the very bodies of the people who live and work within these systems. It is a sad truth that black Americans have long had poorer health than white Americans. They have a higher risk of many diseases, including heart disease, diabetes, and stroke.[11] They also live consistently shorter lives than whites (though this gap has narrowed in recent years).[12] These health gaps are neither random nor inevitable. They are a consequence of history. Centuries of slavery, socioeconomic and political exclusion, and the daily bigotries that emerge from a culture where discrimination remains endemic have all contributed to the poor health of black Americans. These conditions are systemic, with roots in the earliest days of colonization on this continent. If the history of these conditions is the iceberg, then present-day black mortality is its tip.

When we understand how the past informs our present health, we also see how we might engage with historical forces to reverse what hurts us and to improve with what makes us well. This means taking an honest look at the systems that we have built over time, acknowledging their flaws, and working to correct them. Engaging with the past also means recognizing that health is not something that is fixed to a particular moment. It does not happen in an instant, and it is not a result of sudden disease or cure. Rather, it unfolds over time. Our early experiences influence our health throughout life, and our health in turn shapes the health of our children. This argues for improving the conditions that shape health at all stages of life, ensuring that our children inherit the healthiest possible history.

TWO

MONEY

In 1863, with the U.S. Civil War raging, Congress passed the Enrollment Act—the first federal military draft in American history.[1] The Act made every male citizen between the ages of 20 and 45 eligible for Union military service.[2] Enforcement of the draft proved controversial, notably leading to the New York City Draft Riots, the most destructive civil disturbance in the city's history.[3] Anger over the draft was centered on one of the legislation's caveats: the Enrollment Act allowed individuals to buy exemptions from military service for the cost of $300. This led to the perception that the Civil War was "A rich man's war and a poor man's fight" and fueled the anger of the New York City rioters, many of whom were economically disadvantaged Irish immigrants with no money to purchase exemptions.[4]

Economic inequality also shaped the fighting force on the Confederate side: in the South, one exemption was granted to white men for every 20 slaves owned on a plantation.[5]

These are dramatic historical examples, but they're cited here to illustrate a point: money buys health. More than 600,000 soldiers died in the Civil War, whether from combat, accident, starvation, or disease.[6] The power of money and property to secure exemptions, which allowed the wealthy to sidestep the hazards of the war, shows how security and well-being tend to follow affluence.

In the Civil War example, this truth was most fundamentally and brutally expressed in the South. There, those at the bottom of the economic ladder—black slaves—were forced to endure the daily violence of slavery, oppressed by a system designed to secure the wealth and comfort of plantation-owning elites. It is telling that, even during a time of national crisis, when troops were badly needed in both the North and the South, wealth could still provide a buffer between the rich and the dangers faced by everyone else.

The Enrollment Act shows not just how money shapes health, but also how the exercise of federal power can determine who this influence benefits. During the Civil War, a government policy created an opening for money to improve the health of those who already had much. More contemporary policies demonstrate how policy can capitalize on this link and use money to actually improve health. The United States' Earned Income Tax Credit (EITC) is an income-tax credit designed to reduce the tax burden for low-income working Americans.[7] Workers are given a credit that is equal to a percentage of their earnings up to a maximum amount, with both the credit rate and the maximum depending on the size of the family; families with children receive a significantly larger credit than families without children. The EITC has been linked with a number of positive health outcomes, especially for infants and mothers: a 2009 study found that each time the EITC was raised by 10%, infant mortality declined by 23.2 per 100,000 children.[8] Increasing EITC benefits has also been found to reduce rates of low birth weight and to improve health at the neighborhood level by injecting cash into economically distressed areas with high concentrations of low-income families.[9] Just as the Enrollment Act allowed people of wealth to use their money as a shield against danger and disease, the EITC helps mitigate the hardships faced by people who lack the protection that money provides. Both policies illustrate a core truth: whether it's buying safety in a time of war or improving the conditions in which economically disadvantaged mothers give birth, there are few relationships stronger than the link between money and health.

So how does having money improve health? While it is true that those who have a lot of money can afford better healthcare than those who have little, money buys health because it buys access to the conditions that are conducive to heath. Consider education. The United States has a deeply unequal system of public education in which much of the funding for public schools comes from local property taxes.[10] This means that communities with more money can afford greater investment in public schools, and communities with fewer resources cannot. Money also buys access to expensive private schools and higher education. As discussed in the previous chapter, education strongly influences health, shaping the decisions we make, the jobs we can get, and how long we live.

Other health-promoting resources can be bought. Money purchases better food, better neighborhoods, political influence, and, crucially, peace of mind. If a tree falls on your house, money lets you repair the damage. If you need help raising your children, money lets you afford daycare. If you need a break from the psychological stress of work, money lets you to take a vacation. This mosaic of advantage translates into better health.

How does *not* having money undermine health? It makes us less likely to have a decent home in a safe neighborhood, to eat high-quality food, to receive a good education, or to live a long life. The Urban Institute found that the less money a person has, the less likely she is to have paid sick/vacation leave and pension or retirement contributions; a neighborhood with sidewalks, parks, playgrounds, and a library; or to report excellent or very good health.[11] These daily deprivations are challenging enough for an individual; taken together, they represent a cycle of disadvantage that is perpetuated across generations for large numbers of people. For example, people in low-income neighborhoods are less likely to have access to stores that sell nutritious food. This is known colloquially as a "food desert"—a neighborhood where the only available eating options are cheap, unhealthy fare.[12] Food deserts, and the related problem of "food swamps"—areas characterized by a proliferation of fast food—can contribute to obesity in their surrounding communities.[13] Residents of low-income neighborhoods can also face barriers to exercise, including fears of crime, which further exacerbate obesity.[14]

In aggregate, the barriers to health faced by low-income individuals are daunting, even staggering. Living in an area with structural limits on the availability of healthy food, while at the same time being statistically more likely to be undereducated, sick with one of the many chronic diseases that stem from obesity, and/or facing daily racial discrimination—it's a lot. The likely racial discrimination is particularly pernicious, as economic disadvantage is closely intertwined with race.[15] In 2016, 22% of blacks and 20% of Hispanics lived in poverty in the United States, compared with just 9% of whites.[16] Blacks and Hispanics are also likelier to face exposure to more than one of the disadvantages associated with financial instability, including lack of education, lack of health insurance, and living in a low-income area.[15]

For all America's prosperity, the gap is growing between those who can and those who cannot afford the conditions that produce health. In the United States, the richest 1% of Americans now live 10–15 years longer than the poorest 1%.[17] Underlying this trend is an economy in which the distribution of wealth is increasingly concentrated at the highest level. In 2013, 76% of all U.S. family wealth was in the hands of families in the top 10% of the wealth distribution.[18] In 2015, the total retirement savings of 41% of American families—50 million Americans—amounted to $4.9 billion, a sum equal to the total retirement savings of only 100 top CEOs.[19]

As significant as this gap is, it is important to note that when we talk about how economic inequality undermines health, we are not just talking about how it harms the health of people we typically consider to be "the poor."[20] To many, "the poor" means the homeless and the destitute—people we too often consign to the margins of our society. Yet inequality is not a problem of the margins; it touches everyone. This is especially true in the United States, where the bottom 50% of the country has, in recent decades, seen essentially no net increase in pre-tax income even as Americans work longer hours than workers in most other industrialized countries.[21,22] So when we talk about economic inequality, we are talking about half of the people we see every day. That's friends, family, neighbors, selves. And while the core focus of this book is on health in the United States, it is important to remember that the link between money and health is universal. This was illustrated by a staggering 2016 UNICEF report, which found that children born into the 20% of households at the bottom of the global economy are nearly twice as likely to die before *age 5* as those born into the 20% of households at the top.[23]

Accepting that money matters for health means correcting two common misperceptions. The first is that people who lack money somehow "deserve" poor health for not working harder to improve their circumstances. This attitude is deeply rooted in our collective values—especially in the United States. We live in a culture that valorizes the pursuit of wealth, often equating material success with personal virtue. Americans are rapt by a "rags to riches" tale, and we often see that affinity in media— everything from the old stories of Horatio Alger to popular films like *The Pursuit of Happyness* [sic]. However, these stories do not reflect the reality of where most wealth actually comes from. In fact, 35–45% of wealth is inherited.[24] While we may thrill at depictions of the scrappy underdog beating the odds to win his fortune, it is more often a tax code that favors the well-off and their heirs, rather than the indomitable spirit of the individual, and that accounts for most of the millionaires and billionaires in our society.[25,26] In this context, it makes sense that so many Americans continue to face the poor health that comes from financial uncertainty. What does not make sense is our collective insistence on blaming the victims of this system, not the system itself, for this troubling status quo. Our tendency to fault disadvantaged people for the challenges they face reinforces why money is an essential aspect of any conversation about health. When the relationship between money and health is made clear, we can see how disease links to the material disadvantage caused by an economic playing field that is far from level.

The second misperception about money and health is that people with financial means can simply buy their way out of poor health without worrying about the broader conditions that distribute health in society. It is true that for diseases where expensive, cutting-edge medicines can make the most difference, money is a good thing to have. But the influence of money, as important as it is, actually pales in comparison with the larger array of social, economic, and environmental forces that shape the health of populations.

Take cystic fibrosis (CF) as an example. CF is a disease that is highly responsive to the treatments scientists have developed to fight it. In the 1950s, a child with CF stood little chance of reaching her teens.[27] Today, the median survival age for patients with CF is more than 36 years in the United States.[28] In Canada, the median survival age is more than 48 years. What accounts for this gap? It's because the United States, more than any other country in the world, is the most attached to the idea that doctors and medicine can fix all the problems caused by an unhealthy society. So while we spend more on doctors and medicines than does Canada—more, indeed, than any other country—the money and medicine can't uproot the other aspects of our lives that make us sicker. An American with CF is more likely to have a parent plagued by trauma, or be born at low weight, or go home to breathe fumes from the bus depot, or suffer any of the other myriad problems that are inherent to American life, especially if she lives in a poor neighborhood. Money buys health, but it can only buy so much without a proportional investment in everything else that matters for health—in the other 19 chapters of this book.

In acknowledging the link between money and health, we can also see how being healthy means taking a hard look at why some people have money and some do not, then working to reduce the number of "have-nots" among us. It means tackling the conditions of economic inequality and promoting health by pursuing economic justice. In the United States, economic justice would require us to acknowledge, and correct, economic inequities, including an unfair tax code, a system of public assistance that does not go far enough toward addressing the full needs of the poor, and a market-based healthcare law that falls short of providing universal coverage or offsetting costs for all economically vulnerable citizens.

But economic justice does not simply mean addressing existing inequities. It means taking proactive steps to ensure that everyone can afford the resources necessary for health. It means putting money in the hands of people who need it: so they can buy medicines, yes, but, more important, so they can access the conditions that will allow them to live a healthy life. We can do this by expanding the EITC, raising the estate tax and using the revenue to fund public goods, pushing for a single-payer healthcare system and investigating the possibility of providing a universal basic income to all citizens—an idea that is attracting interest around the world.

If we want people to have health, we need to make sure that they have money. This is not a conclusion that Americans have historically been very comfortable with. To many, redistributive economic policies suggest "handouts," taking money from the people who earned it to give it to people who did not, with no clear return on this investment. However, such policies ultimately benefit us all. Putting aside the moral case for caring for those in need, making people healthier by giving them a solid financial foundation also lays the groundwork for our own health.

THREE

POWER

In June 1968, the United States seemed like it was being torn apart by political violence. The assassinations of Robert F. Kennedy and Martin Luther King Jr. occurred within two months of one another, opening wounds that were still fresh from the assassination of President John F. Kennedy earlier in the decade. In the intervening years, the country had been rocked by urban riots, violent crackdowns on civil rights activists, and increasingly militant rhetoric on both ends of the political spectrum.[1] During this tumultuous time, President Lyndon B. Johnson, nearing the end of his time in office and sensing an opportunity to pass legislation that might have been impossible at any other time, chose to address the mounting violence by pushing for reform of the nation's gun laws. After RFK's assassination, Johnson called on Congress to pass legislation that would ban the interstate sale of guns and keep weapons out of the hands of those who might misuse them.[2] In making his plea, LBJ emphasized that "the voices of the few must no longer prevail over the interests of the many." By "the few," he meant the organized gun lobby—specifically, the National Rifle Association (NRA). LBJ was prescient in noting the power of the gun-lobby organization. Despite what seemed like favorable political circumstances for gun safety legislation, the NRA was able to quickly mobilize opposition to the president's efforts, blocking the passage of meaningful reform.[3]

In the years since 1968, America's gun problem has grown. At the time of LBJ's initial call for gun safety legislation, the president cited the yearly average of more than 6,500 gun-related murders in the United States.[4] Today, more than 35,000 Americans die from guns each year, 96 Americans are killed each day, and 25 children die from gun violence each week.[5–7] The proliferation of military-grade weapons has made mass shootings routine, leading to staggering acts of violence in places like Newtown, Orlando, and Las Vegas. In the face of this ongoing tragedy, it is encouraging to find that Americans overwhelmingly favor gun safety: no fewer than 70% of Americans have consistently supported background checks for gun purchases, and 55% of U.S. voters have said that it is "too easy" to buy a gun in this country.[8,9] Support for gun safety is also bipartisan, with 82% of Republicans/people who lean Republican and 85% of Democrats/people who lean Democrat favoring a ban on gun purchases by people on no-fly or watch lists.[10] Despite this broad public consensus, the United States has made little progress on advancing gun safety at the federal level.

The reason for all this is frustratingly simple: public preference and common sense have been blocked by power. A robust majority of Americans support measures to improve gun safety, but a majority of lawmakers who hold the levers of political power continue to oppose such measures. The latter's power has enabled the voices of the few to continue to prevail over the voices of the many. While power can sometimes seem abstract, the gun debate shows how it lies at the heart of the conditions that shape our health and the health of our family and friends.

What is power? The social theorist Steven Lukes has suggested that there are three dimensions of power: overt power, covert power, and the power to shape desires and beliefs.[11,12] *Overt power* is power we can "see." It is characterized by the choices made in public by leaders. It is seen most clearly, perhaps, in executive leadership and in the steps taken by political actors. The use of overt power is often zero-sum, with a certain course of action winning out over the stated preference of others. For this reason, it can be susceptible to reversals, especially when a leader makes a decision without first cultivating a broad base of support, either within her institution or among the public at large. *Covert power* is, by definition, harder to observe and less absolute in its dynamics. It resides in the capacity to set an agenda and work within the complex systems where decisions are often made, using the rules of these systems to control an agenda or otherwise leverage procedure into a desired outcome. Covert power is the power of the committee chair, the parliamentarian, the backroom lobbyist. The *power to shape desires and beliefs* is arguably the subtlest form of power. It relies on persuasion, dialogue, even propaganda, to nudge public opinion toward accepting certain values or agreeing to a certain course of action.

While it may appear less decisive than overt power, the power to shape desires and beliefs can be the most influential over the long term. By working to align public opinion with a particular goal, it can transform notions into movements, shifting culture in the direction of enduring change.

Power shapes health overtly and covertly. Power is wielded in politics, which shape the laws that, in turn, influence the conditions that keep us healthy or make us sick. These are the zoning laws that decide the layout of towns and cities, the agricultural subsidies that decide the ingredients of food, and environmental laws that decide the quality of the air we breathe. Agricultural subsidies, for example, are designed at the political level to promote food availability by making certain commodities cheaper to produce. From 1995 to 2010, the U.S. government spent an estimated $170 billion subsidizing soybeans, corn, rice, wheat, sorghum, livestock, and dairy. These commodities are often turned into unhealthy processed foods, calorie-rich juices and soft drinks, and fattening meat and dairy products. This sea of calorie-dense, nutrient-poor food then engulfs us, setting the stage for unhealthy eating. A 2016 study found a link between the consumption of these commodities and greater risk of cardiometabolic challenges.[13] Political power can subsidize poor health or it can change the existing course by subsidizing more nutritious products like fruits and vegetables.

Power also shapes health by affecting culture, the influence of which trickles down to our desires, expectations, and the social norms we adhere to each day. We like to think of ourselves as independent actors steered by nothing other than our own will. That is not the case. We are influenced far more than we think, and we behave in ways shaped by our society and culture all the time. Power is wielded by figures like the celebrities who set trends and create demand for the products they endorse; thought leaders whose words and ideas advance the public debate; and religious authorities who shape our conscience and beliefs. The importance of cultural power has been evident in a number of social movements, including the struggle for lesbian, gay, bisexual, and transgender (LGBT) rights. In the United States, the LGBT community has made steady progress, from the legalization of gay marriage to the greater cultural acceptance of this long-marginalized group. While the gains for LGBT Americans have culminated in recent years at the political level, they also illustrate the influence of cultural power, as television shows featuring LGBT characters and out celebrities like Ellen DeGeneres laid the groundwork for progress. Former Vice President Joe Biden, whose early endorsement of marriage equality was widely thought to have spurred the Obama administration to greater action on the issue, acknowledged the importance of cultural power when he said, "I think *Will &*

Grace probably did more to educate the American public than almost anything anybody's ever done so far."[14,15] While cultural factors may not seem, in the moment, as consequential as the exercise of political power, their influence over time can be deep and lasting. They change how we think, setting the stage for the laws that then enshrine how we act. Just as changing laws is a key function of power, changing minds is equally critical—and no less representative of how power shapes our world and our health.

How does power work in practice to shape the conditions of health? To answer that question, it is helpful to return to Lyndon B. Johnson, the man who once said, "I do understand power, whatever else may be said about me.[16] I know where to look for it, and how to use it." More than 50 years ago, Johnson signed into law the Social Security Amendments of 1965.[17] These amendments established the Medicare and Medicaid programs, which provide health coverage for eligible low-income Americans and people over the age of 65. The ideas behind these programs had long been a part of the American political conversation and were championed by the late John F. Kennedy. However, by the time of Kennedy's assassination, legislative progress on the issue had stalled. For years, Congressman Wilbur Mills, who served as chairman of the House Ways and Means Committee, had refused to bring Medicare to a vote in the committee, thinking the proposed program to be fiscally irresponsible.[18] When Johnson assumed the presidency, he identified Medicare as a key priority—part of the larger suite of domestic programs that would become known as the Great Society. Initially, Johnson attempted to negotiate with Mills and craft a bill that the congressman would feel comfortable backing. At the same time, Johnson worked to build public support for his political vision, shrewdly using his speeches to tie Kennedy's legacy to his own legislative goals. While the President's initial negotiations with Mills did not bear fruit, Johnson's appeals to the public helped give his Democratic Party the momentum it needed to triumph in the 1964 election, winning sizable majorities in the House and Senate. The Democrats were then able to reorganize the Ways and Means Committee, adding legislators who supported Medicare. Mills saw the writing on the wall and relented, eventually becoming a Medicare ally himself. Mills's about-face had not come out of nowhere: throughout the legislative process, Johnson took pains to gain the congressman's support, calling him regularly and taking him out for meals. LBJ is even said to have joked that he courted Mills with greater care than he had courted his own wife.[19]

The passage of Medicare and Medicaid represents Johnson's skillful use of power in each of its three forms. As a president working in public view to overcome a dedicated opposition and advance change at the federal level, Johnson exercised overt power. By cultivating the support of Mills and using his knowledge of legislative procedure to shape the agenda of a congressional committee he showed his backroom mastery of covert power. By appealing to the idealism of the Kennedy era in order to move public opinion where he wanted it to go, he skillfully shaped desires and beliefs. The result of these efforts was a political victory that, to this day, continues to improve health in the United States.

Johnson's fight for Medicare/Medicaid shows how power can be used "from the top down" to influence health, with federal action creating transformative change. But power can also function "from the ground up," with political actors taking their cues from motivated, highly organized citizens and interest groups. This approach was, and remains, exemplified by Johnson's foe in the gun debate—the NRA.

The NRA has managed to hold the line against safer gun laws for decades by building power along each of Lukes's three axes. It builds overt power through direct engagement with the political process, working to elect candidates whose views align with its philosophy of unfettered access to guns anywhere, any time. It encourages its members to register voters, staff phone banks, distribute campaign literature, and remain politically active and aware between election cycles. Once candidates are in office, the NRA then holds them accountable, giving them a "rating" based on their voting record on guns.[20] The NRA also exercises covert power, working to keep gun reform off the political agenda and undermining efforts to better understand gun violence by influencing the mechanisms of federal funding. In 1996, for example, lawmakers supported by the NRA passed a budget provision saying that no funds allocated to the Centers for Disease Control and Prevention's Injury Center "may be used to advocate or promote gun control."[21] This provision has hindered gun violence research, making it more difficult for those who study the problem to access up-to-date data. Finally, few political organizations have been more effective than the NRA at shaping desires and beliefs. The group has successfully aligned its cause with cherished American notions around individual freedoms, framing any effort to pass more sensible gun laws as an attack on liberty. This portrayal informs all of its activities, turning what was once an organization dedicated primarily to hunting, marksmanship, and conservation into a self-cast champion of freedom—and the powerful political force it is today.[22]

Power also emanates "from the ground up" in less ideological ways, typically in response to injustice or the health needs of marginalized groups. In the example of LGBT Americans, the social and political progress made over the past decade has brought health progress, too: LGBT Americans now face reduced challenges in the areas of hepatitis, substance use, mental illness, and suicide.[23–26] This improvement, in turn, benefits the health of the broader community. The Time's Up movement is another example of this power at work.[27] Founded by powerful women in the entertainment industry to express their solidarity with women facing workplace sexual abuse, Time's Up has successfully raised money to help low-income women access legal defense against sexual misconduct, pushed for legislation to hold companies accountable when they tolerate persistent harassment, and promoted gender parity in the workplace. While still in its early days, the movement represents a multilevel exertion of power to changes culture and the rules that govern our behavior. Campaigns like it have the power to increase equity and health for women and underrepresented groups everywhere.

Thinking about power is essential to thinking about health. In contemporary history, power has been held by people and organizations that actively pursue it and have a demonstrated goal of using it to fundamentally change society. Often these changes are self-serving. Even more often they are not conducive to health. If we do not participate in this pursuit ourselves, with the goal of improving health, others may seize the levers of power to move policies—as well as cultural norms and values—in a harmful direction.

The classic example of this dynamic is the tobacco industry, which wielded its power strategically even in the years before the dangers of smoking became widely known. Through ads and celebrity endorsements, the industry was able to cultivate and insulate a culture of smoking in the United States during the twentieth century. Later, when research had shown the harmfulness of tobacco use, it took decades of data-informed antismoking efforts to challenge the industry's power and shift culture toward a rejection of smoking and its risks. In the meantime, smoking contributed to an epidemic of lung cancer and increased the risk of a range of other health challenges, including asthma and coronary heart disease.[28,29] The tobacco industry built and maintained power by aggressively promoting a narrative that smoking is safe and glamorous. And, by doing so early, they could seize the cultural high ground and hold it for what seemed like an indefinite term. In short, they saw a power vacuum where no one else did and were able to occupy it to promote their own interests. The lesson here is that these vacuums never stay empty for long. They will always be filled—either by those who seek power solely for selfish reasons or those who wish to advance the public good and improve the conditions that shape health. To safeguard health, the latter have no choice but to engage with power.

Power in itself is neither good nor bad. It is a tool, one that can improve or undermine health depending on the intentions of whoever uses it. Robert Caro, LBJ's biographer, once said:

> We're taught Lord Acton's axiom: all power corrupts, absolute power corrupts absolutely. . . . I don't believe it's always true. . . . Power doesn't always corrupt. Power can cleanse. What I believe is always true about power is that power always reveals.[30]

Too often, the exercise of power reveals a desire for profit, for individual aggrandizement, or simply for acquiring more power—frequently at the expense of the conditions that make people healthy. But when justice and a concern for equity lie at the heart of power, it truly can help create a healthier world.

FOUR

POLITICS

More than 2,000 years ago, Aristotle wrote:

> Every state is a community of some kind, and every community is established with a view to some good; for everyone always acts in order to obtain that which they think good. But, if all communities aim at some good, the state or political community, which is the highest of all, and which embraces all the rest, aims at good in a greater degree than any other, and at the highest good.[1]

Health is arguably the highest of all the goods to which we can aspire. Nothing is possible without health; it is a necessary condition for everything else we may wish to accomplish, both as individuals and collectively.

And politics is inseparable from health. Politics is part of the system that distributes the resources that decide whether or not we can live healthy lives—resources like peace, education, economic opportunity, a safe environment, and a just social order. Where politics fails to ensure that all can access these resources, health suffers.

In 2017, we saw this in Yemen, where political instability created the conditions of poverty and war, which in turn laid the groundwork for a cholera epidemic.[2] In Russia, political negligence and the government's deliberate promotion of homophobia have contributed to the largest HIV epidemic in Eastern Europe and Central Asia.[3-5] In the United States, our political failures include continued malpractice on the issue of gun violence and a legacy of economic deregulation that has created a crisis of inequality that undermines the health of millions.

The link between physical and political health has long informed how we think about politics. It is fitting that we refer to a community that lives under a given political system as "the body politic," with political dysfunction often likened to a disease that afflicts this body.[6] This is reflected in literature—extending all the way back to the stories of the Bible—where plague frequently represents punishment for political injustice or corruption.[7] The health of the body politic may even influence how citizens select their leaders. A study of the 2016 U.S. presidential election found that counties with poorer health were likelier to support the insurgent candidacy of Donald Trump.[8] It is not difficult to imagine how Trump's promises to

upend the political system could have resonated with a constituency whose poor health was a product, in part, of the failures
of that system. A community aiming for the highest good must
therefore pursue a healthy politics, with the goal of ensuring
healthy citizens.

The American political conversation is, ostensibly,
dominated by debates about health—from the Affordable Care
Act (ACA or "Obamacare") to the price of pharmaceuticals.
But closer examination reveals that these debates are not actually about health at all. They are about healthcare. *Health* is the
well-being and longevity of people—a reflection of the quality
of the society in which they live. *Healthcare* (and its wonkier
sister term *health policy*) is the system of doctors and medicines
available to sick people. In the United States, we talk almost
exclusively about healthcare.

Politics picks up the slack for our flawed, medicine-centric
conversations about health by legislating and regulating all the
myriad things that mean more to our health than doctors. For
example, traffic safety: it may seem to have nothing to do with
health policy, but the quality of our roads is a critical factor
in deciding whether or not we live healthy lives. It is part of
the broader social, economic, and environmental context in
which we live; a context that is fundamentally shaped by politics. While healthcare is unquestionably important for health, it
is only a small wedge in a much bigger pie—which, at the end
of the day, is what truly makes the difference between health
and disease.

The links between politics and health therefore are many, with politics influencing health perhaps most through shaping policy, public investment, and institutions that keep us healthy. Politics influences everything from the quality of our food and water to the safety of our communities, to the viability of our global climate. In 1999, for example, the Centers for Disease Control (CDC) made a list of 10 great public health achievements from the twentieth century.[9] Among these achievements was motor vehicle safety—an area where health and safety gains have been dramatic. The year the CDC made its list, there were six times as many Americans on the road as there were in 1925, and the number of motor vehicles in the United States had increased 11-fold.[10] At the same time, the number of miles traveled in motor vehicles had increased since the mid-1920s by a factor of 10. Despite these increases, between 1925 and 1997, the annual motor vehicle death rate declined by 90%—from 18 deaths per 100 million vehicle miles traveled to 1.7 deaths per 100 million vehicle miles traveled. What accounts for this decline? Certainly drivers have not changed much in 100 years, nor has the American fascination with the open road. No; the difference was made at the level of politics. In the past century, political actors created regulatory standards for safer roads and vehicles, introduced seatbelt laws, and used safety campaigns to spread awareness of driving laws and best practices.[11–13] Politics also led to the founding of public institutions like the National Highway Traffic Safety Administration and National Transportation Safety Board to monitor and improve the conditions of our roads.[14,15] Through these political measures, we have changed the culture of driving, fostering a safer environment for our travels and saving lives.

Consider, as another example, climate change, arguably the greatest health threat we face in coming decades.[16] Climate change has led to a rise in extreme weather events, which can devastate communities and undermine health, causing mental and physical scars that linger for years.[17] These disasters also cause mass displacement, creating "climate refugees" who often go without medical care and face increased risk of trauma and exploitation.[18–20] And while we are only just beginning to understand the effect that the heat and humidity of a rapidly warming planet will have on future health, early research suggests that the combination can be deadly—deepening inequality between those who can afford shelter from this hazard and those who cannot.[21] The politics of climate change are therefore the politics of health; in the current world, we'll never be healthy (or safe) without tackling climate change at the national policy level. Given that science is unequivocal about climate change's cause (humans) and its pace (accelerating), the main impediment to action is not lack of knowledge: it is a particular political establishment that is committed to denying, downplaying, and, ultimately, worsening this generation-defining health threat.[22,23] Understanding the commercial and political interests that drive this denial, and then countering them in the political arena, are just as important for our health as accessing quality medicines and treatments.

Climate change policy is today's most shining example of the many ways politics affects health without affecting healthcare. Policies and public institutions that foster good—things like equity, affordable housing, better schools, economic opportunity, and global peace—all improve health by creating a place where health can flourish. American history is flush with examples of political initiatives that have illustrated this link: the creation of the Department of Housing and Urban Development and the passage of the Civil Rights Act and Title IX. Globally, international organizations like the United Nations have done the same since the end of World War II. These political successes all contribute to the conditions that allow us to be well and reflect a politics that aims at the highest good: health.

But politics does not shape health through policy alone. Politics also shapes the public discourse, setting the tone of the national debate and influencing the ideas we decide are acceptable for practice or policy. This interplay between ideas and politics is summarized in the concept of the *Overton window*.[24] Developed by the political scientist Joseph Overton, the idea behind the Overton window is that there is a spectrum of options for handling any issue. These options range from the unthinkable, to the popular, to, finally, settled policy. On the side of the unthinkable are ideas considered to be too extreme for the mainstream discourse. On the side of settled policy are ideas that are accepted by the public and codified by the political establishment. Within this spectrum is a narrower range of options—the Overton window—which consist of the ideas deemed fit for the public debate and practicable as policy. Ideas regarded as inappropriate for wider consideration are excluded from this range unless and until the Overton window is nudged in their direction. By voicing ideas on the national stage, shaping media narratives, and exercising the power of office, political actors have the ability to shift the Overton window, moving into the mainstream ideas once regarded as radical or even dangerous.

Over the past 50 years, the Republican Party in the United States has proved particularly adept at shifting the Overton window to reflect an ever-growing disdain for the role of government in American life. In the mid-1960s, the mainstream expression of this view largely reflected a belief in fiscal prudence and the opinion that overregulation stifled the dynamism of the market. Over the years, this view became more extreme, morphing over time into a conviction that government is an insidious, unnatural force whose primary role and utility is in raising and maintaining an effective military. Conservatives accomplished this shift in three key ways. First, they established a scholarly basis for their ideas through think-tanks and academic publications. Second, by engaging with the broader public, they blamed the unrest of the 1960s on the "overreach" of Great Society-era government programs—then used the backlash to that era as a foil for their messaging.[25] Third, they assiduously cultivated political power at the state and national levels, in part through symbiotic relationships with industries lobbying for lower taxes.

Conservative success at shifting the Overton window is seen in the history of the Environmental Protection Agency (EPA), which was created during the administration of Richard Nixon.[26] Nixon was, at the time, considered a very conservative politician. Yet he still acknowledged that government had an important part to play in keeping the environment—and, by extension, the American people—healthy. In his 1970 State of the Union address, he made this position clear: "The great question of the seventies is, shall we surrender to our surroundings, or shall we make our peace with nature and begin to make reparations for the damage we have done to our air, to our land, and to our water?"[27] Despite his ecological sensitivity, Nixon would pave the way for Ronald Reagan, who presided over deep cuts to the EPA and whose famous declaration that "government is the problem" would shape the thinking of a generation of conservatives.[28,29] This philosophy reached a kind of culmination in the presidency of Donald Trump, who attacked the EPA just as aggressively as Reagan, working to cripple the agency through budget cuts and regulatory rollback.[30] In this way, conservative dogma has come to resemble the Ouroboros—the mythical snake who eats its own tail.[31] Republicans have been so successful at shifting the Overton window toward a radical antipathy for the basic functions of government that they see no problem with trying to destroy an agency they helped create—all to the detriment of health.

This is where the American understanding of health as healthcare becomes a problem. As the federal government loudly debates its role as a healthcare provider and facilitator, the bluster masks how political action is shaping health in other ways—specifically, that special interests shift the Overton window toward policies that maximize their own advantage, often at the expense of health. Oil and gas companies seek to do business free of regulation, polluting in the name of profit; Wall Street likewise chafes at regulation, preferring total freedom to pursue wealth, even as economic inequality deepens. This profit motive, which has undeniably led to market innovations that have done much to raise living standards in the United States and around the world, has also led to an entrenched class of permanent interests in this country, creating political conflict between the health needs of the many and the wealth needs of the few.

The tendency of divergent interests to engender conflict was an abiding concern for the architects of the U.S. political system. James Madison tackled this challenge in *The Federalist Papers*, addressing conflict and its implications for the government he was helping to create. He wrote, "The latent causes of faction are . . . sown in the nature of man; and we see them everywhere brought into different degrees of activity, according to the different circumstances of civil society."[32] Madison identified material inequality as "the most common and durable source" of political division. In his era, this manifested chiefly as the "various and unequal distribution of property." In our time, we see this in the unequal distribution of wealth and health. Madison's scheme to mitigate factions and prevent any one group from dominating the rest was to "extend the sphere" of American political life by creating a republic large enough to accommodate a multitude of diverse interests. The sheer range of these interests, Madison reasoned, would prevent any group from becoming too powerful without stifling the healthy debate needed to produce good policy. In this way, the American system was designed to harness the creative potential of political conflict while lessening the risk that it would become destructive.

To overcome the challenge of special interests that work against the conditions that create health, we need to extend the sphere of what we talk about when we talk about health so that our conversation includes factors like money, power, love, hate, culture, the environment, and politics. Good health is in everyone's interest—its constituency includes, potentially, every human being on earth. Activating the political power of this coalition means promoting an awareness of the full picture of what goes into shaping health so that we can see when special interests harm us by undermining our economy, air, water, equity, and more. We can then advocate for health by advocating for a politics that promotes it in every area of American life.

Importantly, we have little choice but to think this way. Without engaging politics to promote health, the conditions that shape health will languish, making our society—and people—sicker. As ever, history shows us what happens when politics becomes disconnected from our thinking about health. In 1848, the Prussian government appointed a pathologist named Rudolf Virchow to study a typhus epidemic in Upper

Silesia, in what is now part of Poland.[33,34] Virchow's visit to the economically disadvantaged region would last only 3 weeks, but the report he produced about his time there would have revolutionary implications. In his report, Virchow painted a picture of social and political dysfunction—of an epidemic aided by poverty, ineffective civil servants, lack of quality education, and other socioeconomic hardships. He concluded, "There cannot be any doubt that such a typhoid epidemic was only possible under these conditions and that ultimately they were the result of the poverty and underdevelopment of Upper Silesia. I am convinced that if you changed these conditions, the epidemic would not recur." To promote health in Upper Silesia, Virchow argued, the people needed education, full employment, agricultural improvement, and other social and economic reforms.[35] The fact that these reforms were necessary in the first place reflected a failure not of medicine, but of politics. Only politics can provide the investment, infrastructure, education, and economic safeguards needed to create a healthy society. If it falls short of these functions, then even the best medicines can do little to safeguard health.

The UN's Universal Declaration of Human Rights, one of the iconic political documents of the past century, states that every individual has a right to "a standard of living adequate for . . . health."[36] The bases for this standard, as Virchow saw, are the socioeconomic conditions, shaped at the political level, that create the context for health in our daily lives. By framing these conditions as a right, the Declaration recalls Aristotle's observation that a political body should aim for "the highest good"—the advancement of health. This is as true for the global political community as it was for the city-states of ancient Greece. To make sure that this right is upheld, we must embrace a political vision that supports the institutions and policies that promote health. It means addressing healthcare and medicine, yes, but, centrally, it means improving the full range of social, economic, and environmental conditions that affect health and are rooted in politics. By doing so, we expand what is achievable within the constraints of our day-to-day political reality while at the same time working to shift the Overton window toward the radical goal of a world where all can live a healthy life supported by healthy politics.

FIVE

PLACE

Sofia is 12 years old. She is playing tag with friends on the street outside her home. The other children are faster than she is, but she refuses to be caught, twisting and turning, weaving between parked cars to escape her pursuers. She can hear the buses pulling into the depot a block away, although she cannot smell their exhaust like visitors to the neighborhood can: she long ago became used to the ever-present reek of diesel. Now she barely notices it, although her mother does, and worries about its effect on Sofia's health. In a few hours, her mother will arrive home from work on one of those buses. It will be late, too late for family dinner. But Sofia will be glad to see her. It has been a good day. She is winning tag.

Then, suddenly, she is not winning. She feels something in her chest, a tightness that was never there before. She stops running and starts to wheeze. Her playmates think she is faking to avoid being "it," until they see her double over. The children do not know what to do, except for one, Luke, whose brother experiences similar episodes. He calls 911 and tells the dispatcher that he thinks his friend is having an asthma attack. Later, when Sofia is recovering in the hospital, a doctor will confirm that the boy was right.

When we last saw Sofia, she was 45 years old and suffering from a number of health issues. Her poor health is the product of the conditions in which she was raised, an interplay of factors that make it difficult to tie any of her illnesses to a single cause. However, for one of Sofia's most long-standing problems, there is a very clear cause. If she had not grown up near a pollution-spewing bus depot, she would likely not have had as many frequent asthma attacks. Sofia's asthma puts her in crowded company. According to the Centers for Disease Control (CDC), U.S. asthma rates increased by 28% between 2001 and 2011.[1] As of 2011, approximately 18.9 million adults in this country and 7.1 million children had asthma. And while the condition's increasing occurrence may give the impression that it's not serious, it is: thousands of children with untreated or exacerbated asthma die every year. It is particularly common among children who are raised in neighborhoods located near major roadways; pollutants produced by traffic emissions are significantly linked to childhood asthma.[2–5]

Sofia's life was shaped by this exposure. Her asthma is a powerful illustration of how surroundings, or place, influences health. "Place" means simply our immediate, day-to-day surroundings. It is where factors like economics, our social environment, and the physical infrastructure of our surroundings coalesce into the space we navigate each day. Place can be a city, a town, a neighborhood, or the overlapping influence of all three. The common link is that place touches our lives daily; deciding what we see, hear, and taste; shaping our health in ways good and bad. If our air is polluted, if our neighborhood is stressful and noisy, if our local market does not carry nutritious food, then it is less likely that we will be able to live a healthy life. If, however, our air is clean, our market supplies an abundance of quality food, and we live in a quiet, low-crime neighborhood, our chance of being healthy is much better. Taken together, the influence of these conditions suggests that our zip code is a better predictor of our health than is our genetic code.

In Sofia's case, place is represented by harmful influences like living near the bus depot, yes, but it is also represented by her community—the network of friends who were there to help her when she fell ill. Her surroundings harmed her, but they also helped her.

The health influence of place can be easy to overlook, in part because it is so close to us. It is like the feeling of air. It touches us always, but we tend to perceive it only when there is a disturbance—when the wind blows. For example, we do not often think much about the quality of our drinking water. But when our water is shown to be unsafe—as it was in Flint, Michigan, for example—we rightly focus on it. Water suggests a further example of how hard it can be to truly *see* what we encounter every day. This example was captured in a story told by the writer David Foster Wallace:

> There are these two young fish swimming along, and they happen to meet an older fish swimming the other way, who nods at them and says, "Morning, boys, how's the water?" And the two young fish swim on for a bit, and then eventually one of them looks over at the other and goes, "What the hell is water?"[6]

Extending the fish metaphor slightly provides a clarifying picture of how place decides whether or not we are able to live a healthy life. Imagine the two fish live in a bowl together, as your pets. You want them to be well, so you feed them the best food, encourage them to exercise regularly, and, when a romance blossoms between the two, provide them with educational materials so that they will know to have safe sex. In short, you promote all of the activities that our culture teaches us produce health in individuals. Then, one day, you wake up to find your fish are dead. What happened? You were so busy making sure that they were learning healthy behaviors that you forgot to change their water.

Place can sustain or limit our ability to be healthy, just as the water in a bowl can keep its occupants alive or sicken them. As humans, keeping our own "water" clean means making sure that where we live supports health on every level. There is no single way that place shapes health—its influence is ubiquitous, and it shapes health through both the physical and social environments.[7] Understanding these conditions may be a first step to improving them.

How does our physical environment (our day-to-day sur-roundings) shape health? Through factors like urban infra-structure, the presence of green spaces, networks of public transportation, and food access. Infrastructure includes things like sanitation, the systems that deliver electricity and drinking water, and the physical safety of the places where we live. When these things are poorly maintained, the health consequences can range from the depression that can accompany living in crumbling, dirty settings to catastrophes like the 2017 Grenfell Towers fire in the United Kingdom, where the outdated design of a public housing block may have helped spread a blaze that left 71 people dead.[8–10]

The Grenfell Towers tragedy is an extreme example of the perils of an unhealthy physical environment. An opposite example—a community that actively fosters mental and phys-ical health—would combine green spaces, infrastructure for ac-tivity (e.g., bike lanes and sidewalks), and accessible modes of transportation that allow residents to get elsewhere safely and cheaply for work and recreation.[11,12]

Mass transportation networks, including bus and train routes, promote health in several ways. By taking us to and from work, they allow us to make the money we need to stay healthy. Transportation also broadens our leisure options; if our neigh-borhood does not have a park, transportation networks help us get to one. Transportation also allows us to pursue educational opportunities by helping us commute to classes.

The component of a physical environment that is arguably most inescapable is its food landscape—the sources of and types of food immediately available to residents. Low-income neighborhoods are often "food deserts," with an abundance of fast-food restaurants and corner markets that carry cheap, processed goods. If the nearest market that carries nutritious food is across the city or in another town, the day-to-day task of maintaining a healthy diet (even for one's self, let alone an entire family) becomes prohibitively daunting.

Of course, place is more than just geography and physical environment. The social environment—the interplay of economic, cultural, and political factors that characterize a community[7,13]—has a sizeable impact. These are factors like labor markets, health services, community institutions, and the local influence of government policies. When these factors are robust within a community, health flourishes. When their influence is weak or nonexistent, it creates the conditions for crime, economic uncertainty, isolation, stress, unhealthy social norms, and, ultimately, poor health. There is a long history of research linking poor heath to an unstable social environment. In 1939, the American sociologists Robert E. L. Faris and H. Warren Dunham suggested that "social disorganization" found in some parts of cities created psychological difficulties among these areas' inhabitants.[14] In the years since Faris and Dunham introduced their theory, data have continued to link frayed social fabrics to undermined health in communities. For example, high concentrations of urban crime have been linked with higher rates of posttraumatic stress disorder.[15] Neighborhood social environment has also been linked with physical health risks, including smoking, obesity, and low birth weight.[16–18]

A healthy social environment produces longer, healthier lives by fostering social capital. Social capital is the network of relationships—both institutional and interpersonal—through which people take care of each other.[19] Social capital can be something as simple as Sofia's friends looking out for her in her time of need. It is the same in our own lives. If we get sick, if we become incapacitated, if we are just under pressure at the office and need someone to look after our kids for a few hours while we work late—we have social capital where we are able to call on a network of friends or on community institutions like our church for assistance. In the best of times, these networks help provide support and meaning in our lives; in moments of crisis, they can be the difference between survival and disaster. The value of social capital was evident after the 2011 Japanese earthquake, tsunami, and nuclear meltdowns, when survivors said that many lives were saved by the actions of neighbors, friends, and family. The social environment is what shapes our access to these networks of support.[20]

In the case of Sofia's asthma, she was fortunate to be diagnosed with a disease that is eminently treatable. There are many effective treatments for asthma to improve quality of life for people who suffer from the condition.[21] Anti-inflammatory drugs such as inhaled steroids can prevent asthma attacks and reduce airway swelling. Bronchodilators can ease asthma symptoms when they arise and be used before exercise—allowing Sofia to return to playing tag. But the existence of these treatments does not change the fact that none of them would have been necessary for Sofia had she grown up in a healthier environment. To return to an earlier metaphor, fish swimming in dirty water eventually get sick.

When we ignore the "water" that surrounds us, or when we are unaware of its impacts, our health will inevitably be compromised; we are in effect putting a glass ceiling on how good our health can be. Medical innovations—as important as they are—can sometimes obscure this fact. Because asthma is treatable, we are less likely to acknowledge how asthma rates are driven by the conditions of place—conditions that we can improve if we choose. Improving these conditions does not just mean ending the practice of putting buildings that generate pollution near residential areas. It means improving the physical and social environment at every level. We see this when we look at the drivers of asthma. In addition to its links to pollution, the disease has been linked to residential segregation, economic hardship, and the social relationships within communities.[22,23] To prevent asthma, we must address all these factors. Doing so can also help us prevent the many other diseases that are associated with an unhealthy physical and social environment. Increased neighborhood social capital has been linked with lower depression rates and with networks of social support helping to improve mental health in communities.[24] Creating healthier places is not just a matter of ensuring that neighborhoods and homes are well designed, that streets are clean, and that the environment is free of toxins (as important as these physical improvements are). It also means making sure everything we come into contact with each day fosters health, including our interpersonal networks.

In 2017, the U.S. Department of Housing and Urban Development (HUD) issued a rule lowering the threshold of lead acceptably present in the blood of children living in federally assisted housing units.[25] The goal was to help the department respond more quickly when these children showed signs of elevated lead exposure, a condition that has been linked to depression, panic disorders, and a range of other health conditions.[26,27] This exposure is powerfully shaped by place: lead can be found in water, paint, dust, soil, and other trappings of a home and neighborhood. By changing its lead policy, the housing department took a step toward improving health by improving the conditions of place. And because place is a ubiquitous variable, HUD's actions on lead represent an example of effecting real change and a powerful tool for promoting health.

All of this is especially true as the world urbanizes. The United Nations projects that, by 2050, 66% of the global population will live in urban areas.[28] Investing in a healthy urban infrastructure; building parks and green spaces; establishing community centers and responsive health systems; building clean, accessible transportation networks; and creating integrated neighborhoods instead of segregating cites by income and minority status—all of these actions can help leverage the influence of place into better health for all.

The conditions of place, however, are not limited to the conditions of a neighborhood. These are likewise the conditions of our world. Global threats like war, poverty, and climate change are the planetary equivalent of dirty water. While we may, individually, think we can insulate ourselves from these threats with wealth or privilege, we all ultimately inhabit the same place— the same global fish bowl. Just as Sofia's health was limited by the conditions of her city block, our own health is limited by the broader social, economic, and environmental challenges that shape life on earth. We cannot escape these conditions, and we have little choice but to work to make them better if we are interested in generating health for ourselves and our children.

SIX

PEOPLE

"Hell," wrote Jean-Paul Sartre, "is other people." The line comes from the play *No Exit*, a drama about the afterlife of three damned souls as they begin their punishments in the underworld.[1] Expecting to face torture for their earthly transgressions, the characters are surprised to find that hell is merely a small room that they must share for eternity. This fate proves more than sufficient as the play unfolds, as the three characters are unable, or unwilling, to provide each other with the mutual support that could help them transcend their situation. The relationships among the characters turn increasingly toxic until they realize, at last, that they are doomed to make each other miserable forever.

Sartre's play captures a key truth: humans are fundamentally social, and our social networks—our often-overlapping groups of friends, family, colleagues, and acquaintances—shape our well-being in profound ways.[2] *No Exit* takes a pessimistic view of this influence, but it is equally true that our relationships can provide the pleasure, satisfaction, and joy that give life meaning and foster health. Where human relationships are nurturing, cooperative, and centered around healthy behaviors, they can be a bulwark against disease. Where they are destructive, or encourage harmful behavior, they can lock us into a cycle of poor health, just as Sartre's characters are locked in their room, sabotaging each other's chances to improve their collective condition. What I take most from Sartre's play is that human existence is inevitably shaped by others, and this extends to all aspects of our life, including our health.

No Exit also captures our shared circumstances as human beings. While we may like to think of ourselves as islands, our biological evolution does not support a life without social networks; in other words, loneliness poses challenges for health.[3] We cannot escape the fact that our well-being will never be a matter of pure self-sufficiency; it is deeply dependent on our interactions with the people around us, the people with whom we share a "room"—our world. To make sure that our world is healthier than the one in Sartre's play, it's essential to talk about people and our place among them.

Human interactions shape health at each stage of life. The first bonds we form are typically with family members who influence our health by taking care of our immediate needs and by modeling the behaviors and values we will carry with us into the world. The next phase of social development is outside our immediate family, cultivating relationships at school, work, and elsewhere. As with family relationships, these friendships influence our values and behavior. If friends engage in risky activities like smoking and drinking, it increases the likelihood that we will do the same. If friends model healthy habits, we are likelier to make these behaviors our own, too. As life progresses, one may choose to have children or to live with a significant other. This represents a further level of social integration, as we become more deeply invested in the networks we have formed over the years. All these stages of social development have a cumulative effect on our health, creating a network of love and friendship that, if properly nurtured, can enrich our lives from youth through old age.[4] Social networks can also improve our odds of *reaching* old age: the more integrated we are into our web of friends, family, and acquaintances, the longer and healthier our lives tend to be.[5]

Who we interact with can also influence the pattern of health and disease among our social networks. This influence is most obvious and simplistic when we talk about contagious diseases. If the people around us are vulnerable to disease—if they are unvaccinated, for example—it increases our own chance of becoming sick. This is so basic that it is easy to overlook— another example of the "water in the goldfish bowl" that we do not notice. Vaccines are a wildly effective tool for mitigating these diseases, but, even then, the effectiveness of vaccines depends on the choices made by the people around us: the more people who choose to be vaccinated, the stronger our collective defense will be; this is known as *herd immunity*.[6] But when the people around us reject vaccination, it undermines herd immunity, and our health can suffer. For example, in the years since measles was declared eliminated from the United States in 2000, a high percentage of measles cases have occurred among intentionally unvaccinated people.[7]

Disease can also spread through our observation and behavior. A 2007 study demonstrated how interactions with other people can be a conduit for spreading behaviors and lifestyles, which in the case of the study was manifested in obesity.[8,9] The scientists evaluated more than 12,000 people over the course of 32 years and found that an individual is 57% likelier to become obese if someone she considers a friend is obese. This link was strengthened if the friendship was considered mutual, in which case an individual's obesity risk rose by 171%. Strikingly, physical distance does not seem to affect the relationship between our friends' weight and our own: the link was found to persist even between friends who were many miles away from each other. This phenomenon is known as *social contagion*,[10] which the *Oxford Dictionary of Psychology* defines as "The spread of ideas, attitudes, or behavior patterns in a group through imitation and conformity."[11] It stems from our tendency to learn by observing and mimicking other people's behavior.[12] Other areas where social contagion may play a role include the spread of smoking, depression, and sleep loss.[13–15]

Social contagion is still a fairly new area of study, but emerging research suggests that it has a profound influence on human health. One study looked at military service members who had been deployed to bases around the United States and found that families of service members deployed in counties with higher obesity rates were likelier to become obese.[16] The risk of obesity was even higher among families who lived longer in a particular location and resided off-base. This study suggests that patterns of health do not just spread through infection; they can also spread through imitation, via our social networks.

While social relationships can aid the spread of bad habits and disease, the lack of relationships can be even worse. We need only look at what happens when individuals are denied access to social networks to see how dependent humans are on the company of others for health, happiness, and survival. Consider the example of long-term solitary confinement, a punishment still in use in U.S. prisons.[17] This practice, in which prisoners are isolated from the prison's general population, can lead to depression, paranoia, hallucinations, and increased suicide risk. But isolation doesn't have to be this extreme in order to undermine well-being; simply being lonely can harm health, too. The mortality risk posed by loneliness is statistically comparable to the hazard posed by drinking and smoking and is greater than the health hazard of obesity.[18,19] In other words, loneliness is a public health issue. In 2018, the English Prime Minister Theresa May acknowledged the scale of this problem by appointing a

Minister of Loneliness to help the country tackle the issue of widespread social isolation.[20]

Long before the United Kingdom chose to address loneliness through the creation of a government office, The Beatles released a song, "Eleanor Rigby," that captured the essence of social isolation—and hinted at its risks.[21] The song's central character, the lonely Eleanor Rigby, is picking up rice in an empty church where a wedding has just taken place. The church is overseen by the equally lonely Father McKenzie, whose job includes writing the words "of a sermon that no one will hear." Both characters inhabit a world that feels indifferent to their isolation. Eventually, Eleanor Rigby dies, and her funeral is tended to Father McKenzie, with no one else in attendance. At the end of the song, Paul McCartney wonders where all the lonely people come from.

The answer to McCartney's question lies with the conditions in society that enforce isolation and disrupt social networks, conditions that include stigma, age, disability, and economic disadvantage. The ongoing U.S. opioid epidemic has shown how stigma can alienate people from one other, isolating those most in need of human connection and exacerbating an arduous affliction. Addiction is a chronic disease that society treats as a crime.[22] We marginalize people with addiction, making it harder for them to reach out to others for assistance. Stigma of similar pervasiveness has contributed to the loneliness faced by individuals in other populations, including LGBT, immigrants, and anyone denied inclusion in their communities.[23]

It is important to note, too, the self-reinforcing stigma of loneliness itself.[24] Because society, particularly American society, places such emphasis on the capacity of the individual to overcome any adversity, it is easy to feel as if acknowledging loneliness is a kind of weakness, a sign that we are somehow not up to the job of navigating modern life. The irony, of course, is that if more people spoke about their loneliness, we could see how common it truly is, reduce the stigma around discussing it, and improve health for all.

Loneliness can also be a product of age and disability, conditions that exacerbate isolation and prevent individuals from engaging with the full life of a community.[25] The problem of loneliness among older people is pervasive: 42.6 million older U.S. adults are estimated to suffer from chronic loneliness.[26] Given that a huge swath of the world's population is about to enter old age, this problem will only get worse if we do not pay attention to it. Already, in countries like Japan, where an aging population has grown ahead of that population in the United States, the country faces the challenge of millions of lonely elderly who experience the health consequences of their loneliness.[27] But loneliness is not just a product of age and disability; it can also make these conditions worse. Lonely adults are likelier to experience mobility declines, difficulty with upper extremities tasks, and difficulty climbing.[28] High levels of loneliness have also been linked with greater risk of physical frailty.[29]

Economic disadvantage is a common source of isolation, confining people to low-income areas and excluding them from the schools, clubs, recreational activities, and jobs enjoyed by people with greater financial resources.[30] This isolation is driven by the globalization that has left many communities behind in the U.S. industrial heartland, even as the other parts of the country reap the benefits of these trends. The people who live in these economically disadvantaged regions face epidemics of addiction, depression, and suicide; these are called "deaths of despair," and they reflect their deepening isolation.[31,32]

In cities, economic disadvantage and the isolation that comes with it is frequently tied with race and residential segregation. In the 1930s, the federally funded Home Owners' Loan Corporation encouraged banks and insurers to approve or deny home loans based on racial criteria, keeping black residents in one part of a city and whites in another.[33,34] Over the years, government agencies also used the construction of public housing units and major roadways to segregate cities, further isolating black communities.[35] As is consistent with U.S. history, this separation was far from equal. Blacks were placed in poor neighborhoods, while whites were housed in more desirable areas, their surroundings less noisy, less polluted, and more conducive to health than the sections designated for people of color. The legacy of this segregation persists. Not only are black Americans likelier to live in economically disadvantaged areas, but even affluent black families are likelier to live in poorer communities.[36] In the United States, 37% of black families earning $100,000 or more per year live in poor areas, compared to just 9% of white families.[37] This combination of place, race, and economic vulnerability fuels isolation, excluding many black Americans from the full range of privileges enjoyed by their white counterparts.

All these factors compound contemporary isolation in an era when cultural and technological currents have made it all too easy to slip into loneliness. In many ways it has never been easier to imagine that we can exist without face-to-face human interaction: digital devices let us consume vast quantities of entertainment whenever and wherever we want, social media is reshaping our communications, and powerful drugs appear to offer an escape hatch from life's challenges—though, as the opioid crisis makes painfully clear, this seeming escape hatch is actually a deadly trap door.[38] These conditions have the potential to keep individuals more isolated and unhealthy and prevent them from seeing the conditions that underlie their loneliness. It's the core tragedy of "Eleanor Rigby"—not that its two characters are lonely, but that they are lonely *so near one another* without ever connecting. Vexingly, and like Sartre's characters in *No Exit*, Eleanor and Father McKenzie have the potential to provide each other with the compassion and support that could dramatically improve their circumstances. But, for whatever reason, they do not. It reflects the challenge of building healthy social networks in the twenty-first century. Our technology keeps us intimately linked while also pulling us apart. Like Eleanor and Father McKenzie, we are alone, together.

As much as we may like to think otherwise, we are not islands. And until we address the conditions that undermine our social networks, health will remain poor. To build this world, we must invest in common spaces where communities can come together and strengthen social ties—from public schools, to community centers, to safe injection facilities where people with addiction can go without fear of stigma. It also means making cultural, religious, and civic institutions as inclusive as possible. Consider the social and health victories that have followed the U.S. Supreme Court ruling in favor of same-sex marriage: it struck a blow against isolation, allowing gay Americans to access the social stability, legal protections, and health benefits that come with marriage.

Finally, we must acknowledge, out loud, the widespread existence of loneliness and its effects on health, helping to destigmatize this very common condition. It means creating structures that support people at times in their life when they are likeliest to be lonely, and it means creating communities that are more inclusive of older adults and people with disabilities. Home visits, mentoring partnerships, and exercise programs can all help to keep older adults socially integrated. Providing physical accommodations and the universal health coverage necessary to meet the needs of the disabled can go far toward ensuring that they can remain engaged members of society.

At the end of the day, talking about health means talking about people—and making sure that people are talking to each other. Human contact within social networks can be an incubator for social movements; social movements can build a healthier world. For example, the HIV/AIDS movement, which has saved countless lives by advancing better ways of preventing and treating the disease, emerged from the networks of marginalized, largely LGBT people who, at the start of the epidemic, had few people willing to advocate for them in the broader society. By banding together and finding allies in the United States and around the world, these activists managed to overcome the loneliness imposed by stigma and disease and make remarkable progress against HIV/AIDS in just a few decades. Similar community-based movements have made progress in gender equity, environmental justice, and civil rights.

Health is only improved when people leverage community networks on behalf of the common good. Our individual health and our capacity to build a healthier world are rooted in the quality of the social networks we develop throughout life. Or, to put it more simply (and revise Sartre), "Health is other people."[39]

SEVEN

LOVE AND HATE

After the September 11, 2001, terrorist attacks, New Yorkers circulated a poem that spoke to the city's pain in the weeks following the tragedy.[1] Named for another infamous date, "September 1, 1939" was composed by W. H. Auden to mark the date that Germany invaded Poland, an act of aggression that sparked World War II.[2,3] Evoking the battlefield with its line, "The unmentionable odour of death / Offends the September night," the poem is unsparing in its analysis of our human capacity to hate and destroy each other. On the threshold of global war, it looks toward the coming years and concludes that, faced with such peril, "We must love one another or die."

Auden well understood the power of hate and the redemptive necessity of love. His poems chronicle both—from the

institutionalized hate found in political repression to the am-
orous love of romantic partners.[4-6] It is no surprise, then, that
when the world was on the verge of a second world war, the
poet would turn again to love, this time to frame it as the only
alternative to ruin. In the wake of 9/11, when it looked as
if the forces of hate once again had the wind at their backs,
Auden's case for love took on renewed relevance.

But what does this have to do with health? We seldom think
of love and hate as linked to health, but they are central to
the issue. In the early days of World War II, and later in the
immediate aftermath of 9/11, hate threatened health in stark
terms: imminent threats of violence through acts of war. Love,
meanwhile, served as a path to building the resilience needed to
withstand the dangers of the moment.

But love and hate do not need a time of crisis to shape
health; they influence our well-being every day. Hate creates the
trauma and divisions that undermine the health of individuals
and societies. Love functions as the antidote, fostering acceptance and community and the health benefits that come with
them. As history has shown, both love and hate mobilize people
in pursuit of ambitious goals that can shape society in ways
both positive and profoundly negative. In World War II, hate
led to the deaths of millions and the crime of the Holocaust.
In South Africa, after the end of apartheid, love was on display
during the country's Truth and Reconciliation Commission, as
family members of apartheid's victims sought justice for their
murdered loved ones.[7] Their testimonies helped the country

process the injustice of its past and transition into a new political era without the violence that can accompany such shifts.

The forces of love and hate are in continual conflict. This
is regularly dramatized in popular culture—from the light
and dark sides of the Force in *Star Wars* to the battle between
Harry Potter and Lord Voldemort. Popular culture defines
love and hate by their mutual opposition, with human actions
manifesting both sides. Given to hate, humans strengthen its
ability to undermine health by creating a society that welcomes
anger, bigotry, and violence. By embracing love, humans can
achieve a healthier society, one characterized by compassion,
solidarity, and respect.

Individuals choose between love and hate each day in their
interactions with other people. Collectively, we choose between
love and hate in the political sphere. The acuity of this relationship was on display in August 2017, when a group of white
supremacists marched on the city of Charlottesville, Virginia,
to protest its intent to remove a statue of the Civil War General
Robert E. Lee.[8] The protesters saw Lee's efforts to preserve
the "right" to own slaves as a gallant defense of a racial hierarchy worth returning to. Their beliefs, and their presence in
Charlottesville, inspired a counterprotest composed of people
who stood against the tide of bigotry and hate.[9] The encounter
between these groups eventually turned violent, and a young
woman named Heather Heyer was killed when a man who
sympathized with the white supremacists allegedly drove his
car into a crowd of counterprotesters.[10] Just as the conflict in

Charlottesville was inflamed by the hateful message of the white supremacists, the tragedy was deepened by the equivocating rhetoric of President Trump. In his comments on the violence, the President hesitated to condemn the white supremacists, saying instead that there was bigotry and violence "on many sides" that day.[11] These events show how hate does not exist in a vacuum; it emerges from our politics and the complex system of forces that define health and society.

How does hate shape health? The events in Charlottesville reflect how hate undermines health through three pathways: (1) by threatening people's physical well-being through violence and trauma, (2) by destabilizing communities through bigotry and hateful rhetoric, and (3) by laying a foundation for political policies that embed hate in the laws and institutions that structure our society. This makes hate (and love) very much part of the complex ecosystem that makes up the "water" of our health.

I have spent much of my career studying the first of these pathways—the health consequences of traumatic events—and have come to see trauma very much as one of the fundamental consequences of hate. Trauma is "an emotional response to a terrible event like an accident, rape, or natural disaster," and it is an experience that can have a profound, lasting impact on an individual's health.[12] The victims of violence in Charlottesville joined the many Americans who experience such trauma each year. More than 199,000 Americans die annually from injuries and violence, and more than 90% of the population experience trauma at some point in their lives.[13] Each minute, 20 people are victims of violence committed by an intimate partner; one in two women (and one in five men) experiences sexual violence in her lifetime.[13] In the United States, easy access to guns amplifies hate's potential to cause trauma, as we have seen in the frequent mass shootings that menace our society. The health consequences of trauma include depression, posttraumatic stress disorder, and higher risk of substance use—all of which can continue to shape health for years after the traumatic event occurs.[14] Trauma suffered in early childhood, for example, is strongly linked with alcohol dependence later in life.[15]

Hate also harms health through the words it can provoke. The saying "Sticks and stones may break my bones, but words can never hurt me" may offer some consolation, but it's fundamentally untrue. In fact, words can cause trauma. Perceived discrimination has been linked with greater mortality risk among older adults, suggesting how the experience of bigotry can accumulate in a person's psyche, undermining health.[16] Hate speech also harms health by dehumanizing it targets, creating the conditions for social exclusion and violence. We saw this in the violence in Charlottesville, in both the rhetoric and symbols used by the white supremacists, including their chants of "Jews will not replace us" and their adoption of fascist symbols.[17–19] These proud proclamations of intolerance were in keeping with larger shifts toward a freer expression of hate in the public conversation in recent years, shifts that have roughly coincided with the political emergence of Donald Trump.

Since his arrival in politics, Trump has proved adept at shifting the Overton window toward an ever-greater acceptance of bigotry and hate as standard elements of public discourse. He began his presidential campaign by targeting Mexican immigrants and Muslims in shockingly overt terms; he later refused to immediately reject the endorsement of white nationalists, and he has continued to encourage, and engage in, racially suggestive hate speech during his time in office.[20–22] That the person holding the highest office in the country—arguably in the world—would talk this way has accelerated and amplified the chorus of hate in the United States, giving greater license to incidents of bigotry and exponentially harming health.

Hate's third pathway to undermining health runs through the politics that codify hate in the systems that shape our society. This kind of politics has had a long life in the United States. Our political history begins with the assertion that "all men are created equal," but even as these words were written, a system of enslavement was in place to ensure that black Americans could not share in this promise or even be counted as citizens of the country they were forced to help build.[23,24] And, were it not for this system, there would have been no slavery for Robert E. Lee to defend, no reason for his admirers to march on his behalf in Charlottesville. Politically informed conditions like segregation, Jim Crow laws, voter suppression, and the economic disenfranchisement of black Americans all emerged from the originating injustice of slavery and our failure to fully reckon with it.[25] This failure has allowed hate, at key points in our national past, to be metabolized into law, shaping (and endlessly harming) the well-being of the people these laws affect. The legacy of race in the United States shows how hate can influence all the forces we have discussed so far that matter for health—from the past, to place, to power, to economic structures.

But, as powerful as hate is, it can be overcome, as has been seen throughout history when people have mobilized against it. This was clear in the week following Charlottesville, when it appeared that demonstrators sympathetic to the white supremacists in Virginia planned to hold a similar rally in Boston. While they succeeded in holding the rally, their turnout of approximately 100 people was eclipsed by an estimated 40,000 counterprotesters who assembled to champion tolerance and respect ahead of hate.[26] Trump's anti-immigrant rhetoric has also been met, at nearly every turn, by louder voices welcoming those who would make the United States their home. His actions catalyzed a surge of activism on behalf of immigrants, notably in the protests that occurred in airports across the United States after he signed an executive order banning immigration from certain Muslim-majority countries and in sweeping rallies following his separation of children from their families on the southern border.[27] This response points to how love can inform the social movements that lead to a healthier, more just society. From black Americans' struggle for civil rights to the fight for marriage equality, effective social movements have long embraced love as an organizing principle for building a better world.

Love, in the context of these movements, does not mean simply love between individuals—romantic love or the love of a parent for a child. It means an unwillingness to tolerate injustice, disease, or pain among anyone, anywhere. This feeling is known as *agape,* or unconditional love for humanity that is not tied to the hope of gain.[28] It is an active love that seeks to do good and improve conditions for all. In his 1958 essay, "An Experiment in Love," Martin Luther King Jr. defined agape as "[U]nderstanding, redeeming good will for all men. . . . It is an entirely 'neighbor-regarding concern for others,' which discovers the neighbor in every man it meets."[29] King's words recall the Christian tradition in which he was raised, a doctrine that calls on its adherents to "love thy neighbor as thyself."[30] But agape is not tied to any specific religion or spiritual belief. Whenever people act on behalf of others by seeking to make the world better for them, they put this love into practice.

Our poor health is inextricably linked with a history of hate and exclusion that has produced societal structures that make us sicker. Accordingly, we have no real choice but to reject hate and embrace love's potential to shape a better society—if for no other reason than the alternative, hate, hasn't worked. One of these manifestations of hate, residential segregation, continues to harm people: segregation has been linked to an estimated 176,000 deaths each year.[31] Segregation also shows how hate can lead to the partitioning of resources away from marginalized and minority populations—deficits that are then exacerbated by factors like power and politics. Charlottesville was a moment that forced us to confront hate in all its ugliness and to see how easily it can lead to injury and death. Yet hate's deepest harms do not generally occur in broad daylight on a crowded street. Hate is rarely so overt.

Hate in the United States is often as subtle as it is systemic, manifesting in social, economic, and environmental conditions that inform and degrade life for millions of Americans. Countering hate means more than simply rejecting it, just as building a better society means more than simply declining to make the status quo worse. As Saint Augustine wrote:

> Do not imagine that you love your servant when you refrain from beating him, or that you love your son when you do not discipline him, or that you love your neighbor when you do not rebuke him. This is not love, it is feebleness. Love should be fervent to correct.[32]

Love that is "fervent to correct" the injustices that underlie poor health reveals itself in action. It pushes to dismantle the structures that allow hate to spread and to build new ones that safeguard health by ensuring an equitable distribution of the resources that produce it. It is unafraid of identifying and "rebuking" the socioeconomic misalignments that undermine health, even when doing so may be unpopular or incur the opposition of powerful interests. It embraces the collective good while understanding that this may sometimes entail individual sacrifice.

When the world looked like it was hurtling toward catastrophe, the poet Auden proposed love as a counterweight to the
forces of hate and self-destruction. More than 70 years after
World War II, some might imagine we have left crises of that
magnitude safely in the past. However, the conditions that undermine health in our society—from the opioid epidemic, to
segregation, to the treatment of immigrants, to the threat of
gun violence—do so on a scale equal to the mortality caused
by some of history's deadliest conflicts. These hazards are often
helped along by hate.

In the face of these insidious challenges, Auden's words continue to ring true. It may be that the struggle between love and
hate will go on indefinitely; that hate is ineradicable from our
nature and will be a source of division and harm as long as
our species exists. If this is to be the case, then to stay healthy
we must remain attuned to the power of love—and perhaps
the wisdom of poetry—heeding especially another famous ex-
hortation of Auden, one of which King and Augustine would
surely have approved: "You shall love your crooked neighbor /
With your crooked heart."[33]

EIGHT

COMPASSION

*I*n the capital city of a great kingdom lived two friends. One was a poor blacksmith who shared a tenement in the city's slum with his wife and children. The other was a rich man, a counselor to the Queen. The rich man pitied his friend and tried to help him when he could. He gave the blacksmith money without asking for repayment and lent a sympathetic ear when the blacksmith talked about the challenges of living in a poor neighborhood. Poverty in the slums was deepening by the year. Worse, there were rumors of a disease of some kind spreading among the overcrowded tenements.

The counselor was a busy man. With his energy invested in court affairs, it never occurred to him to lobby the Queen to help the slums. They were just a few city blocks, after all; a small part of a vast kingdom. The residents' problems were real, but they were relatively minor in the grand scheme, and did not diminish the broader trajectory of the realm, where overall living standards were improving dramatically.

The counselor also knew, in his more reflective moments, that his own comfort and well-being made the problems of people like the blacksmith seem somehow less urgent to him. Like everyone at court, he had access to the best doctors and medicines; these advantages made it easy to feel like health was a readily available commodity, and the problems of the slums could be contained by the great advance of progress. Whenever he felt guilty about his complacency, he gave his friend more money, eventually insisting on paying for the education of the blacksmith's children.

One day when the two friends met, it was clear that the blacksmith was gravely ill. The slums were in the midst of a full-blown epidemic; even the blacksmith's son had begun to show symptoms. The counselor was horrified. He gave his friend all the money he had on him and promised to come back with help. He ran to the Queen, who consented to the use of her personal physician. The counselor returned to the slums with the doctor, but there was nothing they could do. The blacksmith died. The counselor returned to court.

A few days later, the Queen developed a cough. Her illness gradually worsened, until it became clear that whatever had infected the slums had now infected the sovereign. Soon, the Queen was dead. As the country faced a crisis of leadership, the counselor tried not to think about who might have carried the pestilence into the throne room.

This story is an example of what can happen when we think poor health is someone else's problem, or that a health threat seems far removed from our own reality. The counselor, even with his firsthand knowledge of the conditions in the slums, still believed that money, power, and medicine were enough to provide a barrier to disease. He saw health as a commodity, something he could purchase for himself and for the people he cared about. In doing so, he failed to reckon with how his friend's illness was linked to the broader conditions of the slums—conditions the counselor had the power to influence and improve. Instead, he decided that providing charity was as far as his reach extended and that it would be enough to make a difference.

This story makes the case for *enlightened self-interest*, a philosophical concept that posits that helping others is ultimately helping one's self. By helping the slums, the counselor could have saved his queen. Because he did not recognize how his inaction threatened the realm, the tale ended tragically. Yet there is more to the story than this perhaps too-tidy moral. Yes, the counselor might have saved the Queen by helping the slums. But her death was by no means certain. It is possible that the slums could have grown sicker and sicker without ever infecting the monarch. Does this mean that the counselor had no reason to take action after all? It does not: he might have acted because it would have been the right thing to do. He might have acted from a sense of compassion.

According to one dictionary, *compassion* is "sympathetic consciousness of others' distress together with a desire to alleviate it."[1] Compassion is the bridge between the suffering we experience as individuals and the suffering experienced by others. It reminds us that there can be no relief for the individual without improving the structures that underlie the collective. To return to the words of Martin Luther King, Jr.: "True compassion is more than flinging a coin to a beggar; it comes to see that an edifice which produces beggars needs restructuring."[2]

Compassion, then, could be seen as the difference between mourning the loss of one black woman who dies in childbirth and mourning the shameful fact that black mothers die at three to four times the rate of their white counterparts during childbirth (a disparity driven by a range of factors, including racism and socioeconomic disadvantage).[3] Compassion urges us to correct problems like these, even if they do not seem to affect us directly. It links our engagement with the conditions that shape our health to the values that shape our conscience, a refusal to un-see injustice, inequity, and the poor health they produce. In his book *On the Basis of Morality*, eighteenth-century German philosopher Arthur Schopenhauer argues that morality itself stems from "the everyday phenomenon of *compassion*, . . . the immediate *participation*, independent of all ulterior considerations, primarily in the *suffering* of another, and thus in the prevention or elimination of it."[4] Compassion is not about what harms us, but about what harms others and what we choose to do about it. To quote Schopenhauer again, "Only insofar as an action has sprung from compassion does it have moral value."[4]

This is an uncompromising, even uncomfortable, statement. After all, we all have many worthy motives. *Empathy*, in particular, allows us to imagine ourselves "in the shoes" of another person, helping us to "feel" their suffering, and perhaps inspiring us to help. Yet Schopenhauer suggests that only compassion can motivate an act of moral value. This speaks to the difference between compassion and empathy.

Empathy opens us to the experience of others. It prompts us to consider what it would be like to face challenges such as homelessness and hunger, to be afflicted with a life-threatening disease, or to be marginalized because of economic status or skin color. It was empathy that motivated the counselor to give money to the blacksmith, and empathy motivated the Queen to send her personal physician to help a suffering subject. Empathy is what whispers in our ear, "it could happen to you," inspiring us to show people in distress the same kindness we hope they would extend to us in our hour of need. It is this reciprocity that informs the Golden Rule, "Treat others as you wish to be treated."

Compassion improves on empathy. It is not about treating others well so that we may be treated well in turn; it is about us treating others well because that is how they should be treated. It does not imply reciprocity; it aspires to do good for its own sake. Compassion envisions, and aspires to, a better world where collective well-being is everyone's responsibility. In so doing, compassion nudges us to see beyond the individual and recognize the social, economic, and environmental conditions that are responsible for her suffering. Because, until we recognize these forces, the healthier world that compassion urges upon us will continue to elude us. This is what makes compassion a cornerstone of our quest to create a healthier world.

Empathy, alas, is a poor substitute for compassion. If we accept empathy as sufficient, we risk thinking we are creating a healthier world through altruism alone, when, in fact, what we leave in place are the structures that create disease. The counselor convinced himself that giving his friend money and sympathy compensated for refusing to improve the conditions of poverty and neighborhood disadvantage that led to the blacksmith's distress. In these actions, we see how empathy, when it is anything other than a prelude to compassion, can distract from the steps that improve health for all. Reducing poverty or investing in healthier neighborhoods would have improved conditions for the blacksmith and then could have saved the slums, and the Queen, from deadly disease. Instead, the counselor settled for providing charity, which, while certainly a kindness, does little to create a world where charity is not needed in the first place.

The United States has a long history of embracing empathy while stopping short of the compassion-informed action that can truly safeguard health. This is particularly evident after natural disasters, like the string of hurricanes that devastated communities in the summer of 2017. Americans are consistently empathetic after such events, mobilizing quickly to give money and time to assist relief efforts, doing much to help people whose lives are devastated by disasters.[5] However, the key to a community's resilience does not lie with how it responds after the damage is done, but with the condition of a region in the years leading up to the calamity. When Hurricane Maria struck Puerto Rico, it revealed how economic disadvantage and a weak infrastructure can amplify the damage caused by a storm.[6] These challenges slowed recovery on the island, compounding the humanitarian costs that are still felt long after the storm. A compassionate approach would be investing in building resilient communities long before a large-scale catastrophe occurs—a sort of "anticipatory compassion" that could help us preempt the worst of the suffering after disasters. This is worth pursuing, not because we are personally threatened by every natural disaster that occurs, but because we shouldn't live in a world where millions are exposed to needless, preventable risk.

Empathy similarly falls short in the wake of gun violence, especially after the mass shootings that now characterize American life.[7] When these shootings occur, it is common to hear people in positions of power express empathy, typically in the form of "thoughts and prayers" to the victims and their families. While such expressions are of course entirely appropriate following such tragedy, political figures often insist on emphasizing "thoughts and prayers" in lieu of any effort to address the structural causes of gun violence—namely, the nation's lack of common sense gun laws, such as universal backgrounds checks and a ban on assault weapons. This protocol of public empathy has done much over the years to ensure that Congress takes no meaningful steps on gun safety reform.

By showing us the interdependence of the conditions that shape health, compassion also shows us just how much of our health comes down to luck—from the circumstances of our birth to the socioeconomic status of our parents. The Queen, for example, was born into her role, just as the counselor also likely came from a privileged background. Meanwhile, the blacksmith's children, through no fault of their own, faced a narrower range of options in life due to their unlucky origins. Compassion urges us to help them, not out of some grand altruistic impulse, but because we understand how the same conditions that make them sick could just as easily undermine our own health. The saying is indeed true: "There but for the grace of God go we."

At heart, there can be no health for all without compassion for all. Health depends on public goods that are sustained by people who may never use those goods but who nevertheless pay into the system, driven by compassion. When we invest in public goods—better neighborhoods, quality education, and economic policies that specifically benefit people who struggle financially—we create the conditions for health to flourish at all levels of society. Without compassion, we are likelier to be swayed purely by self-interest and disinvest from the public goods that promote health. This dynamic has unfolded steadily since the 1980s, when the United States began reducing its investment in many of the social safety net programs and public institutions that protect the well-being of its citizens.[8] In this time span, the United States has fallen gradually behind its peer countries on nearly all key health indicators despite spending more on health than any other country in the world. Why? Because we have de-emphasized compassion in our public policy. When we weaken environmental protections, make Medicaid harder to access, refuse to raise the minimum wage to a livable level, and encourage economic exploitation by deregulating the financial sector, we are saying that we do not care about the circumstances of others—that, as far as the court is concerned, the slums can fend for themselves. No amount of medical innovation or individual charity can offset the harm this backsliding has caused. To regain the ground we have lost, we have little choice but to return to the sense of collective responsibility that initially inspired a robust American investment in health-promoting public goods. Americans must use the levers of power to institutionalize compassion and commit to helping others, regardless of whether or not we help ourselves in the process. Because it is the right thing to do and because the national future requires it.

Compassion is what makes humans human. It reminds us of our shared vulnerability to the broader conditions that shape health. Compassion also urges us to rethink the moral calculus we use to determine who gets help in our society and what form that assistance takes. This is especially needed in the United States, where social vulnerability is stigmatized and poor health is regarded as a consequence of poor decisions or an underdeveloped sense of morality. We see this attitude in those who talk of "the undeserving poor" in discussions of federally funded welfare programs or who imply that certain groups "deserve" disease due to their "lifestyle." Compassion helps us widen our ethical lens and see how sickness has nothing to do with morality, but that morality has everything to do with whether or not we tolerate the conditions that make sickness more likely among particular populations. Helping these groups means moving beyond expressions of empathy or isolated acts of charity to tackle the true causes of their poor health. This in turn helps us all.

NINE

Knowledge

For thousands of years and across multiple human civilizations, the pursuit of health was guided by the theory of *humorism*.[1] This theory, which originated in ancient Greece, proposed that health and disease are shaped by four bodily fluids, or "humors": blood, yellow bile, black bile, and phlegm. These humors were thought to be linked to the four elements of fire, water, earth, and air, respectively. According to the theory, health depended on keeping the fluids balanced; too much of a given humor was believed to produce physical and mental disorder. Fevers, for example, were thought to be the result of an excess of blood.[2] The cure for this supposed excess was to drain the body of the humor until balance was restored. This led to the acceptance of bloodletting as a common medical treatment, which was widely in use from the days of Ancient Egypt until the nineteenth century.[3]

We now know that bloodletting is extremely dangerous and that humorism is, in a word, nonsense. This is not to say that the doctors who believed in humorism and its associated remedies were foolish or acting in bad faith. It simply means that their actions were constrained by the limits of what they knew.

What we know about health is shaped by the questions we've asked and scientifically tested to date; these questions are as broad or as narrow as our knowledge allows them to be. If we believed that humorism is what governed health, we'd push at the boundaries of how we understand that framework to understand it more fully. (Significantly, this type of inquiry is what helped us recognize the fault of thinking in humors.) If we think that doctors and medicine are the only factors that shape our health, it makes sense that we would only ask about how to cure ourselves if we are sick, even while failing to ask what we can do to stay healthy in the first place. To this end, it's worth considering what we mean when we say that we "know" something—and whether it's worth considering what we don't know.

Epistemology, the study of knowledge, suggests that knowledge is the sum of three parts: truth, belief, and justification.[4,5] *Truth* means that, for knowledge to be authentic, it must be true. *Belief* is clearer cut: it's our truth, however untested or unjustified it might be.[6] It would not make sense to know something while at the same time not believing it.[7] The third criterion for knowledge, *justification*, is the more difficult piece. Plato's dialogue *Theaetetus* says that knowledge is "justified true belief."[8] It's not enough to merely believe something; that doesn't make it knowledge. We must be prepared to provide evidence to back up our claim. Evidence comes from the systematic analysis, which in the context of health and science is embodied in the scientific method.[9] Using the *scientific method*, which entails rigorous testing of a hypothesis and continual reexamination of findings, belief is either justified or it is found to lack the empirical basis of true knowledge. This process is indispensable for creating the policies and practices that foster health.

This road to knowledge is rarely a straight line. Rather, it's a process of continual exploration and refinement, entailing debate, delay, and retraced steps. As the history of humorism shows, knowledge generally emerges after long periods of trial and error; better understanding emerges by standing on the shoulders of those who came before us. This path to knowledge may at times seem convoluted, but its destination justifies it in helping society move beyond what is just belief.

The outputs of the scientific method face different paths out in the real world. Sociologists Uri Shwed and Peter Bearman have suggested that there are three trajectories for a belief on the road to knowledge—whether it's "justified" as true or arrives at a more ambiguous outcome.[10] The first is called a "spiral" trajectory. According to Shwed and Bearman, this is when "substantive questions are answered and revisited at a higher level." This is a fundamental aspect of the pursuit of knowledge: questions beget more questions. The more we know about something, the more we see how much we still have to learn. A spiral trajectory occurs when we have answered the basic questions in a line of inquiry and then begin to tackle the more nuanced puzzles that emerge from our early conclusions. For example, we know that income is closely linked to health. We also know that this link is influenced by factors like the quality of the food, education, healthcare, and general opportunity that money lets us access. These basic questions are answered, so now research can start to address the subtler shades of this influence: the correlation between growing income gaps and growing wealth gaps in the United States, the role of poverty in deepening poor health, and the like.[11]

The second trajectory is the "cyclical trajectory"—when "similar questions are revisited without stable closure." This is what happens when researchers fall on two sides of a possible conclusion with no resolution in sight. In contemporary science, we see this in the debate over the population health effects of salt. There is little question that too much salt adversely affects health for those with high blood pressure or other heart conditions. The stickier question is whether, by reducing salt consumption in whole populations, including for mostly healthy people, we will improve health. This debate has raged in the field for decades. A 2016 analysis of 269 reports on salt (of which I was an author, in full disclosure) found that 54% supported the hypothesis that reducing population salt intake is good for health, 33% contradicted that hypothesis, and 13%

were inconclusive.[12] Our study also found that both types of papers—those in favor of the salt hypothesis and those opposed it—mostly cited papers that echoed their findings. This is a classic example of a cyclical trajectory: scientists have "taken sides" and are not speaking across the aisle. And so the salt debate continues, and our knowledge of salt's health influence on populations remains inconclusive.

The third trajectory is called a "flat" trajectory; it occurs when "there is no real scientific contestation." This is the path of most of society's core scientific knowledge, including scientists' acceptance of Bernoulli's principle that slow-moving liquids and gasses create more pressure than fast-moving ones—a phenomenon that serves as the basis for airplane flight.[13] Its universal acceptance is reflected in the nonexistent debate over whether or not planes can fly, not to mention the lack of congressional debate over whether airplanes are safe.

French sociologist and philosopher Bruno Latour suggested that when scientific consensus has been reached—when we are able to say we "know" something is true—the conclusion can then be considered a "black box."[14] The metaphor of the black box, borrowed from the world of cyberneticians, means that when a machine system is especially complex, a black box can be used as a shorthand to indicate that all that is needed to know about it, for functional purposes, is its input and output. Latour points to the workings of a computer as an example of a black box. While most computer users are not familiar with the full workings of their device, they need only really know the machine's input and output—how to turn it on and how to enter and extract data—to use it successfully. A well-made scientific conclusion assumes a similar kind of functionality. It is something that works, that we can depend on as the basis for future study and for the practical measures that can improve our world and our health.

Latour's progressive, perhaps overly optimistic, approach has not been in line with how science has been received by the general public in recent years. We live in an age when scientific knowledge is routinely politicized, belittled, and dismissed by those in positions of power. Consider the conflict over climate change. The science of climate change is unambiguous: the earth is warming, the process is accelerating, and humans are the cause. This threat is imminent and growing, and yet climate change, which amounts to nothing less than an existential threat to our shared future on this planet, has become a partisan issue in the United States. Republicans overwhelmingly either deny the existence of climate change or misrepresent our scientific understanding of it, suggesting even that there is "debate" where in fact there is none. (Democrats—and, for that matter, the vast majority of governments and political leaders around the world—acknowledge the seriousness of climate change and seek to address it, albeit with varying degrees of passivity.) There are many reasons for the divide on this issue, from the political clout of the oil and natural gas industry to the strong currents of polarization in our society. Regardless of the cause of the rift, climate change exposes a key fault line between facts and everyday life: no matter how secure we are in our knowledge, politics and ideology can effectively "veto" our capacity to implement changes for the betterment of health.

However different the applications of knowledge may be, and however politics may play a role in suppressing or accelerating this application, why does all this matter? Why does our approach to knowledge need all this context? Because, ultimately, we want to understand what causes health. And if we have an incomplete understanding of what produces health, this pursuit is liable to take wrong turns. For example, we have accepted the link between health and diseases. We accept the power of medicine to cure sickness. But we have yet to fully accept how our broader circumstances are an equally powerful influence over our health, even as our knowledge of this influence has grown. Our acceptance of diseases as a threat to health spurred us to develop drugs and vaccines to protect ourselves from epidemics; we've taken no equivalent steps around how health is cultivated from our surroundings, and our national conversation has not fully translated the knowledge we have into meaningful action.[15,16] To be truly healthy, we must understand what produces health, follow where the data lead, and then be clear-eyed about enacting the measures that address these forces. If we do this with the same vigor reserved for, say, taking antibiotics when we have an infection, there's no limit on where society can go from here.

On this there is cause for optimism. Despite the barriers that are often imposed between knowledge and its effective application, history teaches us that facts are resilient, that they can be abused and suppressed but never eliminated, and that, over time, they tend to win out. For evidence, look to the steep decline in U.S. smoking rates.[17] Smoking was once ubiquitous in this country, bolstered by the tobacco industry's marketing prowess and successful infiltration of cultural norms. While these efforts succeeded for many years in encouraging cigarette use, dishonest marketing could not change the fact that smoking kills. An industry (or political entity) can only traffic in non-truths for so long before people begin to notice.[18] When the facts about smoking became more widely known, smoking rates began to fall. This awareness was catalyzed by the 1964 report of the Surgeon General's Advisory Committee on Smoking and Health.[19] The landmark report communicated the dangers of smoking in clear, data-driven terms, cutting through the distortions of the tobacco industry and laying the groundwork for decades of progress against cigarettes. By capturing the public's attention, and alongside a wave of pushback against the tobacco industry, it also showed how facts can make for the most compelling marketing, especially when the data are well-presented and serve an honest narrative.

To reproduce the tobacco effect on other fronts in the pursuit of health, we need the best possible data so that we will have a knowledge base on which to proceed. In light of disinvestment from this approach in the United States, we are well short of having that data right now: in a 2016 report from the Centers on Disease Control (CDC) on the nonmedical factors that influence health, the best available data were a decade old and did not paint an up-to-the-minute picture of how these factors shape our health.[16,20] Our knowledge of these conditions is caught in the middle of a "spiral" trajectory— we know enough to be certain about the link between health and social conditions (housing, money, power, politics, transportation, racial injustice—the topics in this book), but we do not yet have all the facts we need in order to answer the next tier of questions about the nature of this influence. How, for example, will better transportation networks save lives? What is the full health impact of expanding the Earned Income Tax Credit? How much would it cost to capitalize on the health value of cash transfer programs and establish a universal basic income in the United States? Answering questions like these means investing in the production of knowledge, both in the academy and across the sectors that generate data about the conditions that shape health. It means shifting resources away from our overwhelming focus on the development of new medical treatments and toward research that deepens our understanding of how our lives' contexts influence our health. If we do not improve our knowledge in this area, we will neither be able to improve our health nor counter the misinformation that threatens the public's awareness of the true causes of disease.

In the eighteenth century, a new medical procedure emerged that would, over the years, inspire passionate condemnation in moral and religious terms. George Bernard Shaw called it "a particularly filthy piece of witchcraft."[21] To others, it was "no longer medicine, but for the most part destruction," and "forcing . . . dead corruption into the blood of children."[22] The procedure was vaccination, and the pushback it inspired is evidence that even the most revolutionary health advances can face a crucible of fierce opposition. While vaccine skepticism remains with us, immunization has gained widespread acceptance for a simple reason: it works. But vaccination's proven health benefits are not the only reason that the procedure has endured. It has also done so because political leaders—from Thomas Jefferson to United Nations Secretaries General—have heeded the data on vaccines and worked to promote their use.[23,24] As a result, vaccination has saved countless lives, eradicated smallpox, and is on the verge of eradicating polio.[25,26]

When it comes to health, there is no alternative to facts. Reliable, evidence-based data are the foundation of the conditions that keep us well. Building our knowledge of the social, economic, and environmental factors that shape health and applying that knowledge to the improvement of these conditions could improve health as seismically as the advent of immunization. To find out, we must strengthen our science and broaden our understanding of how the forces covered in these chapters link to our health.

TEN

HUMILITY

He is terribly rare. He is like Bach, who in his time had a great concentration of ability, essence, knowledge, a spread of music. Astaire has that same concentration of genius; there is so much of the dance in him that it has been distilled.[1]
—George Balanchine

Fred had an ability to surmount form, and to seem to create at the same instant a new form, which is the mark of an intrinsic dancer.[2,3]
—Martha Graham

I remember when I was doing a film with Fred Astaire, it was nothing for him to work three or four days on two bars of music. One evening in the dark grey hours of dusk, I was walking across

the deserted MGM lot when a small, weary figure with a towel around his neck suddenly appeared out of the giant cube sound stages. It was Fred. He came over to me, threw a heavy arm around my shoulder and said: "Oh Alan, why doesn't someone tell me I cannot dance?": The tormented illogic of his question made any answer insipid, and all I could do was walk with him in silence.[4]
—Alan Jay Lerner

It may be that no one knew more about dance than Fred Astaire (with the possible exception of Ginger Rogers, who, it has often and appropriately been said, did everything Astaire did, only backward and in high heels).[5] His iconic film, television, and stage performances revolutionized how movement could be used to express emotion and drive a narrative. His influence extends from Gene Kelly to Rudolf Nureyev.[6–8] Even the fight scenes of Jackie Chan owe some of their kinetic brilliance to Astaire.[9] Of all the dancers and choreographers who have been exposed to Astaire's artistry, the only one who seems not to have been impressed by it is Astaire himself. Where others saw mastery, Astaire appears only to have seen what he did not know. He was keenly aware of (what he imagined to be) his limitations, and his virtuosity was informed, always, by deep humility. He understood too well the constant possibility of error, and the nagging feeling that, no matter how proficient one becomes, there is always more to learn.

Astaire's self-doubt shows us how humility is, in its own way, an essential part of knowledge. His career embodies the paradox faced by all of us who seek to understand something, whether it's dancing or the conditions that shape health: the more we know, the more we realize how much we do not know. The only way to transcend our limitations is to have the humility to acknowledge that they exist. As the American historian Gary Wills wrote in his mediation on Socrates:

> Continual questioning came, for Socrates, out of a continual *need*, a *lack* of knowledge. Only the thirsty person is desperate to drink, only the person needing love will go out to seek it. . . . That is the paradox of intellectual leadership. It must come from a sharp perception of the *absence* of knowledge.[10]

In the preceding chapter, we talked about how knowledge and understanding are critical for the creation of health. Here, we will talk about why humility, and recognizing what we do *not* know, is just as important to the pursuit of health. As we have seen, this pursuit provides many reminders of how little we know. We are still learning, for example, about the health effects of various chemical exposures, about the causes of addiction, and about the many ways our context shapes our health.[11] We have made profound errors, including humorism, even as we have deepened our knowledge of the structural forces that influence our well-being. As our understanding of these forces has improved, we are constantly reminded that they are complicated and that our knowledge of them will always be, to some degree, incomplete.

It is with due humility, then, that we can embrace the idea that the business of generating health is bigger than the steps any one of us can take to make ourselves healthier. Our well-being is interdependent: I cannot be healthy if you are not healthy, and the conditions that affect you could soon affect me. So, while our understanding of what causes health points us to new ways to improve these conditions, humility helps us resist thinking that progress is inevitable or that we already know all we need to know in order to bring about change. Humility helps us learn. While knowledge may be subject to limitations, humility shows us where the boundaries are, so that we might continually stretch them, widening our understanding of the forces that shape health.

Humility is more than modesty or self-effacement. Humility is rooted in an awareness of forces greater than ourselves—forces that interact within a complex system to shape health.[12] This interaction can produce an effect that is greater than the sum of its parts, influencing health in ways that can be difficult to understand. If, for example, a neighborhood suffers from violence, crime, and dilapidated infrastructure, the combination of these challenges creates a new influence, one that is distinct in itself and in light of its parts. In systems science, this is called *emergence*; that is, the property of a system that is separate from the properties of its components. Health is one such emergent property. (Recall Sofia, whose health was the product of the sum total of her circumstances, not any one factor.) The scale and complexity of this type of influence argue against simplistic explanations of disease, the kind that consider only how isolated causes produce isolated effects. Humility helps us see how limited our understanding often is, especially in the face of all we still have to learn about this complexity.

In their study of the psychological implications of humility, psychologist Jennifer Cole Wright and her colleagues described the core of humility as:

> [T]he understanding and experience of oneself *as one* . . . as a finite and fallible being that is but an infinitesimal part of a vast universe, and so has a necessarily limited and incomplete perspective or grasp on the "whole," which is infinitely larger and greater than oneself.[13]

Fred Astaire was not humble because he truly felt he could not dance—if that had been the case, he would have stopped performing. He was humble because he understood the medium of dance to be much larger than the talent of any one individual, even one as gifted as he was. Astaire was grounded in a sense of his own fallibility. In medicine, doctors make a pledge to practice with humility, the spirit that is articulated in the first words of the Hippocratic oath: "First do no harm."[14] By committing to this principle, doctors acknowledge their potential to undermine health through overreach or error. They recognize that, for all their learning, what they know will always be dwarfed by what they have yet to discover. For this reason, to be effective, they need humility.

Humility is an acknowledgment that the world is shaped by forces bigger than we are. Health likewise depends on others, just as Fred Astaire's performances depended not just on skill, but on the directors, technicians, actors, and dance partners who populated his professional habitat. Our health is not just about us—our diet, how much we exercise, and the like. It is about the people and forces that surround us and the complex interplay of these factors.

Do we really need humility to recognize this? Isn't the history of health a history, in large part, of increasingly sophisticated medical breakthroughs triumphantly saving the day? Are not these breakthroughs evidence that we *can* innovate our way out of any sickness? It is easy to think like this in light of all the advanced drugs and technologies and new treatments developed seemingly by the day. But the reality is that these treatments can only do so much in the face of the broader conditions that shape health. Consider the challenge of HIV/AIDS prevention, an area where we have made much progress in just a few decades. Since the early days of the HIV/AIDS crisis, prevention has evolved from condoms and sexual education campaigns to the use of powerful medications like Truvada, a drug which, when taken daily, is 90–99% effective at preventing the spread of HIV.[15] This is science at work.

But, despite the existence of such drugs, HIV is nowhere near eradication. The virus continues to undermine health around the world, especially in South Africa, where 7.1 million people live with the disease.[16] The South African HIV crisis is the largest such epidemic in the world, and it is occurring at a time when we could prevent all cases of the disease if we perfectly applied what we know. This is evidence of how even the most cutting-edge medicine is not sufficient, on its own, to create a healthy society.

HIV persists in South Africa because a complexity of factors keeps it there. In the presence of these factors, knowing what transmits HIV is not enough to stop it. Actual progress would mean understanding the structural factors that continue to promote disease: the poverty, stigma against LGBT populations, and the marginalization of sex workers that we allow to happen even as we work hard to develop better medications. These are factors we understand only obliquely, and so the epidemic of a preventable disease persists. Solving the problem of HIV means, first, having the humility to recognize that even the most effective drugs will not be enough to eradicate it if we do not tackle the conditions that allow it to flourish.

Humility can also save us from the acts of sheer folly that can occasionally characterize and derail the pursuit of health. These acts generally occur when we take steps based on faulty data, with our confidence stronger than our evidence. In the nineteenth century, mainstream opinion held that disease was caused by "miasma," or "bad air" produced by sewage and rotting matter.[17] When a cholera epidemic struck London, the miasma theory led many to believe that the disease was transmitted through the air, when, in fact, it spread through drinking water that had been contaminated with feces.[18] While germ theory had not yet been proved (because there were no microscopes then capable of seeing bacteria), the pioneering epidemiologist John Snow believed there was a connection between cholera and the city's water supply. However, he faced an uphill battle to gain acceptance for his idea. As the debate raged between Snow and those who believed miasma was causing cholera, valuable time was lost and hundreds died from the disease.[19] Eventually, Snow was able to trace the spread of cholera back to a single water pump on a London street.[20] His argument was not enough to make the scientific establishment let go of its miasma theory. While germ theory would win the day in the long run, the example of miasma shows just how long it is possible to cling to a bad idea, even in the face of contradicting data and dire circumstances.

This type of overconfidence, or hubris, is what happens when humility does not inform our pursuit of health. Hubris is an excess of pride in one's own capacities, and its presence can blind us to the larger forces that shape health and put our well-being at risk. Hubris is an archetypal theme of myth and literature—from the fall of Icarus to the pride of John Milton's Satan in *Paradise Lost*. It is often associated with scientific pursuits—a rather dark reflection of the spirit of discovery that motivates our quest for knowledge. In Christopher Marlowe's play *Doctor Faustus*, for example, the eponymous character is portrayed as a scholar who reaches the limits of earthly knowledge and then is driven by hubris to sell his soul to the devil in exchange for otherworldly powers.[21] In Robert Louis

Stevenson's *The Strange Case of Dr. Jekyll and Mr. Hyde*, Henry Jekyll is a doctor whose hubristic belief in his own abilities leads him to scientifically isolate the worst elements of his nature in the form of an alter-ego, the evil Mr. Hyde.[22] And in Mary Shelley's *Frankenstein*, the protagonist, Victor Frankenstein, believes that science can help him conquer death itself.[23] His hubris causes him to create a tormented, murderous creature whose existence ultimately brings only pain.

In these fictional accounts of scientific and medical pursuits taken too far, the consequences of hubris are grotesque, tragic, and seemingly farfetched. Characters like Jekyll and Frankenstein make for compelling drama, but their ego-driven risks in the name of personal discovery could never reflect our own priorities, could they? In the United States, our health spending suggests that, in fact, it already does. The United States pours money into the development of increasingly more costly treatments at the ongoing expense of improving the conditions that truly shape health. In doing so, we show our willingness to wager our health on the power of medicine and to ignore the deeper forces that make our world the way it is. Our 2011 study that traced deaths in the United States back to the influence of these nonmedical forces unearthed stark data: 245,000 deaths in the year 2000 could be attributed to low education; 176,000 to racial segregation; 162,000 to low social support; 133,000 to individual-level poverty; 119,000 to income inequality; and 39,000 to area-level poverty.[24] These deaths were all products of the complex forces that shape health. Humility helps us to see this and to recognize how, to save lives, we must engage in the difficult, sometimes tedious work of improving these conditions. Yet hubris tempts us to accept these deaths as simply "the way it is"—a price to be paid until the day inevitably comes when we have finally found a cure for everything.

Our faith that medical advances will ultimately save us has blinded us to the real-world consequences of this belief: each time someone dies from a condition like poverty, low education, or racial segregation, they are dying from our collective hubris. By investing all our resources in the promise of medicine rather than the improvement of conditions that shape health, we tell ourselves that future progress is worth present misery, thereby begetting more misery. Humility exposes the fallacy in this choice. It recognizes the limits of keeping ourselves healthy through medicine alone and reminds us that, if we are to improve health, we must improve the conditions around us.

When we take a humble approach to health, we are better able to serve the marginalized groups for whom humility is not a choice. For those of us lucky enough to have access to money and privilege, these circumstances afford us the luxury of sometimes losing sight of that. Because, as long as our luck persists, as long as our own health feels like it is in good hands, we can indulge the belief that conditions do not matter. This isn't an option for people who lack quality healthcare, who live in poverty, or who suffer from any of the other forces that quietly, insidiously undermine health. For them, humility is enforced by the conditions in which they live. They know too well how their health links to these conditions, how irrelevant and distant the advance of medical progress feels compared to the immediate health effects of lacking money or an education or a stable social network. As long as anyone is cut off from the conditions and resources that foster health, everyone is at risk. Any argument to the contrary is just hubris.

ELEVEN

FREEDOM

It is an emblem of Freedom. It was lovingly carried on the battlefields of Germany and France, and on the Pacific Seas and Islands. . . . It will never be furled as long as men of courage are willing to fight and die for the rights and freedoms guaranteed them in the Magna Charta [sic], in the Declaration of Independence and in the Constitution of the United States and especially in the Tenth Amendment thereof which reads: "The powers not delegated to the United States by the Constitution nor prohibited by it to the States, are reserved to the States respectively, or to the people."

These words well summarize how many Americans feel about their flag. The flag symbolizes freedom, recalling a rich history of events and ideals that gave birth to our democracy. The Declaration of Independence expresses these freedoms at their most aspirational; our Constitution enshrines them into law. Together, these documents form the basis for our "experiment in self-government."[1] While our system is by no means perfect, generations of Americans have decided that it is worth defending, that the meaning of the flag is a noble cause around which to rally. This sentiment underpins the attachment Americans feel to freedom and helps explain why the defense of freedom is so central to our national narrative.

The trouble is, the stirring words quoted above do not refer to the Stars and Stripes. They refer to the Confederate Battle Flag, the symbol of an attempt to destroy our democracy and void its aspirations by denying freedom to millions of black Americans. The quote comes from a 1957 article in *United Daughters of the Confederacy* magazine, which attacks the U.S. Supreme Court's ruling, in *Brown v. Board of Education of Topeka*, that racial segregation in U.S. schools is unconstitutional.[2–4] The article specifically invokes the Tenth Amendment to argue that school desegregation "usurps" states' rights, infringing on their freedom to regulate education as they see fit. In the article, the fight against desegregation is portrayed as a continuation of the Southern struggle for "freedom" during the Civil War—specifically, the freedom to disenfranchise and exploit black Americans.

This definition of freedom demonstrates how challenging it can be to understand what freedom means. As much as we think we understand it and as it dominates our discourse and political soundbites, it remains, as a concept, quite nebulous, subject to wildly different, emotionally charged definitions. For as long as America has stood for freedom, there have been people who have interpreted this freedom as a license to do everything they wish, even if it harms others. To *United Daughters of the Confederacy* magazine, freedom meant being able to live at the top of a racial hierarchy that marginalized black Americans. To Civil War secessionists, it meant freedom to profit from slave labor.

Fortunately, the freedom to own slaves and institutionally segregate society are no longer acceptable exercises of freedom in the United States. But the fact that they once were illustrates how freedom can pose such a systematic challenge to health. The injustices of slavery and segregation represented extreme forms of prioritizing maximum individual freedom over health, privileging the well-being of white Americans at the expense of their black counterparts. We continue to tolerate less egregious but still harmful cases where freedom for one person can mean poor health for another.

Individual freedoms in close proximity to one another are bound to produce conflict. Should one person's freedom allow him to smoke near your kids or pollute your drinking water to maximize his company's profits? Should I be able to buy an automatic weapon with ease and carry a concealed weapon into a school? These all represent one understanding of freedom. But are they good for health? Unquestionably they are not. So what about when our freedom puts our own health at risk?

The contradictions inherent in the American idea of freedom—this tension between maximizing individual freedom and protecting the well-being of citizens—reflect how our understanding and application of freedom is a central determinant of our ability to live safe, healthy lives. Freedom matters for health, but for its effect to be a positive one, those freedoms must not infringe on others' rights to life, liberty, and the pursuit of happiness. Whether we choose to prioritize maximum individual freedom at all costs, regardless of the health consequences, or adopt a more nuanced view of freedom, one which values the ability to live free from disease as much as it values an individual's freedom to do as she wishes, will determine how healthy we are at liberty to be in our society. In the 1860s, the conflict between two different understandings of freedom—the freedom to own slaves and the freedom to not be one—led to a destructive war. Today's attitudes toward freedom continue to shape life and death by shaping the policies we pursue to promote health—from gun safety reform to smoking bans—while at the same time motivating much of the opposition to such measures.

American freedom has long evoked images and notions of "rugged individualism," in particular the archetype of the cowboy. In popular mythology, the cowboy is portrayed as a tough, capable loner who takes care of himself. He does not need help from anyone, certainly not from the clumsy hands of Washington politicians. This ideal is informed by the individual liberties suggested in our founding documents and in America's history of westward expansion, which saw generations of pioneers seek the space to pursue happiness on their own terms on the country's frontier. According to this mythos, Americans thrive most when the individual is given a chance to succeed or fail according to her own initiative, free of undue constraints. This belief has informed everything from the debate over school choice to the backlash against the Affordable Care Act—particularly the individual mandate initially included in the law—to efforts to regulate possession of the object so central to the cowboy image: the gun.[5–7] In each of these contexts, the argument for individual liberty has been a potent political tool, helping to block efforts to expand the role of government in the lives of citizens, even when such expansion might improve health.

In the United States, the argument for individual freedom is so powerful that it need not even be applied to individuals to be effective. In recent decades, it has been used in the political arena to hinder federal regulation of corporations and spur broad disinvestment in the public goods that were designed to promote health. Individual liberty was core to Ronald Reagan's political philosophy and to his administration's policy of scaling back investment in the structures that promote health in the United States; as we have discussed elsewhere in this book, this disinvestment has done much harm over the past 30 years. This trend began with Reagan's mission to get federal government "off the backs" of citizens so that individual freedom might flourish.[8] Not surprisingly, it was during the Reagan administration that the United States started seeing a gradual rollback of the gains it had made on health in the preceding decades.[9] American health has fallen behind that of its peer countries since the mid- to late-1980s, coinciding with a period of government disinvestment in the resources needed to create environments that create health. Our promised freedom to do what we want has meant, in practice, that we have become saddled with poor health that robs us of individual and collective freedom to pursue happiness.

It is fitting that Reagan's signature image was one of a cowboy—from the ones he played in his Hollywood days to the Western imagery of his political career.[10] His rise to power was, in many ways, a perfect synthesis of the mythology surrounding frontier-inspired individualism and its real-world political effects. By linking the cowboy spirit to a vigorous program of deregulation and spending cuts, the "Reagan Revolution" undermined many of the core institutions and policies that safeguard health in the United States.

The irony is that the cowboy myth on which Reagan's political activity was based is, itself, based on a misreading of history. The settlers of the American West, for all their hardiness, did not "tame the frontier" without help. In fact, they received significant assistance from what many of their descendants would decry as "big government." A large number of these settlers were beneficiaries of the Homestead Act, an 1862 law that allowed any American adult citizen to claim up to 160 acres of nearly free public land, provided that the citizen agreed to live on the land and cultivate it.[11,12] Ultimately, more than 1.6 million claims would be approved under the Homestead Act, with the final claim approved in 1988.[13,14] The law's longevity shows how even the Americans we today regard as models of rugged individualism were at first willing to accept government help when they understood that doing so was in their best interest.

The success of the Homestead Act is, in some ways, a paradox. On one hand, it is a clear example of the government taking an action that seems to preempt individual initiative. Rather than give people the freedom to merely fend for themselves on the frontier, it created a rough kind of safety net, guaranteeing Americans a piece of land they could call their own if they were willing to make the often-perilous journey west. On the other hand, by providing the basic necessity of land, the Homestead Act paved the way for greater individual liberty, empowering Americans to build new lives however they saw fit. (This freedom came at the expense of indigenous populations' freedoms, as they were threatened, displaced, and often killed by American continental expansion.)

The Declaration of Independence and the Constitution give Americans fundamental rights of citizenship and provide a legal structure designed to maintain these rights. Proponents of unfettered individual freedom often argue that these rights alone are sufficient for Americans to live happy, healthy lives. In this view, the purpose of government is to uphold these rights as they are written and otherwise keep out of the peoples' affairs. However, by offering Americans land and the opportunities that come with it, the Homestead Act acknowledged that the government has a broader role to play in promoting the well-being of citizens. It did so not only by safeguarding their rights, but by maximizing their enjoyment of these rights by providing access to basic public goods.

Just as the Homestead Act carved out space in the wilderness for Americans to thrive, measures that expand access to the resources that promote health in our own time can likewise create space in our society for greater freedom. This alternative view of American freedom, one founded on collective investment in widening access to the resources that enable a healthy life, is part of a larger tradition in the United States, one that is just as enduring as the individualism-at-all costs ethos. This tradition was eloquently captured by Franklin Delano Roosevelt in his 1944 State of the Union Address.[15] In the address, FDR called for a "Second Bill of Rights," which he regarded as essential for the well-being of U.S. citizens and the maintenance of global security. The proposed new rights included the following:

> The right to a useful and remunerative job in the industries or shops or farms or mines of the Nation;
>
> The right to earn enough to provide adequate food and clothing and recreation;
>
> The right of every farmer to raise and sell his products at a return which will give him and his family a decent living;
>
> The right of every businessman, large and small, to trade in an atmosphere of freedom from unfair competition and domination by monopolies at home or abroad;

The right of every family to a decent home;

The right to adequate medical care and the opportunity to achieve and enjoy good health;

The right to adequate protection from the economic fears of old age, sickness, accident, and unemployment;

The right to a good education.[15]

These rights link directly to the forces described in this book, the forces that shape health. Education, employment, a safe and secure living environment—all these conditions are core to our well-being. They also inform a kind of freedom that is both descended and distinct from the rights to "life, liberty, and the pursuit of happiness." Rather than simply guaranteeing these foundational rights, they also guarantee the means to achieve them, offering a blueprint for the correct way for us to think about freedom with respect to health. These are examples of "positive rights"—rights grounded in a collective commitment to ensuring, through public policy and investment, that everyone can access the resources they need to truly pursue a happy, healthy life.[16] Absent any such commitment, our freedom rests on "negative rights"—rights that do not require the provision of resources, only the assurance that individuals can act as they wish, with minimal outside interference. FDR, for his part, regarded positive rights as the natural and necessary evolution of the freedoms expressed at our country's founding:

This Republic had its beginning, and grew to its present strength, under the protection of certain inalienable political rights—among them the right of free speech, free press, free worship, trial by jury, freedom from unreasonable searches and seizures. They were our rights to life and liberty.

As our Nation has grown in size and stature, however— as our industrial economy expanded—these political rights proved inadequate to assure us equality in the pursuit of happiness.

We have come to a clear realization of the fact that true individual freedom cannot exist without economic security and independence.[15]

Individual freedom also cannot exist without health; this truth is, to use a relevant phrase, "self-evident." We cannot do what we wish to do if we are sick, and we cannot be healthy without access to the rights FDR prescribed—rights to social, economic, and environmental conditions that shape well-being. Where these conditions are suppressed in the name of preserving individual liberty, people are reduced in the long run by opening the door to disease and preventable harm. American insistence on total individual freedom has led us to invest too little in the policies and institutions that promote health, undermining our well-being and diminishing our freedom. Because of this failure, our health, compared to that of our peer countries, is mediocre. And it means that, for all our justifiable pride in the rights for which our flag stands, the United States is, in fundamental ways, less free than countries whose citizens enjoy better health.

When our concern for freedom is only applied to the narrow interests of the individual, it too often means that others are free only to be sick and die young. True freedom comes with accepting modest checks on what we can and cannot do, with the understanding that these limits will help safeguard the health of all. At the heart of this acceptance is an essential largeness of spirit, a willingness to make minor sacrifices to serve the greater good.

Such measures are especially important for the health "have-nots" in our society, those Americans who suffer most from our failure to improve the conditions that surround us. When we promote health by investing in public goods—environmental protections, quality education, universal health coverage, a fairer economy, laws designed to promote health and safety—it benefits everybody, maximizing well-being and, with it, the freedom that comes with being able to live a healthy life. However, these benefits are exquisitely important for people whose health is already tenuous as a consequence of living in a society where, more often than not, we neglect positive rights in the name of individual liberty. When we improve the quality of our schools, for example, by investing in public education rather than by simply creating more charter schools, it is particularly meaningful to students whose opportunities are limited by factors like racism, economic disadvantage, or lack of social capital even while it benefits all Americans. While de-emphasizing school choice in favor of broader investment in public schools may limit individual freedom to a degree, it is only through such investment that we can maximize opportunity for all students, with particular benefits for those whose options in life would otherwise be limited by their circumstances. This opportunity translates into health, which in turn means freedom.

Freedom, the saying goes, is not free. This statement is usually applied to the sacrifices made by the military personnel who place themselves in harm's way to defend our country. But there is a second meaning suggested by these words. Freedom is also not free in the sense that, in order to truly exist, it requires our collective investment in the conditions that create health in our society. Health is what allows us to live the promise of our country's founding documents. And, without investing in it, the aspirations of these documents will remain just words on a page.

TWELVE

CHOICE

Every day, we make choices that affect our health. We choose the food we eat, the amount of exercise we get, and whether or not we engage in risky behaviors like smoking, drinking, or unsafe sexual practices. In addition to these daily decisions, we make life choices that influence our health over the course of many years. We choose who to marry, where to live, and our profession. These choices shape income, social networks, and the physical space we inhabit, all of which profoundly influence our health, as we have discussed in previous chapters.

When we make these choices, from the momentous (choosing a spouse) to the mundane (choosing breakfast), we believe that we are choosing freely. We imagine our choices to be, for the most part, beyond the reach of outside influence and that, when we choose, we do so from an unlimited array of options: no one tells us what to eat, whether or not we are permitted to exercise, or who we must embrace as a life partner. For this reason, much of our conversation about health has to do with "lifestyle"—making the correct choices for ourselves, choices which, we believe, will lead to better health.

But are our choices really as unfettered as they seem? Can we really choose to be as healthy as we want to be? To answer that question, let us turn to a perhaps unexpected authority.

The film *The Devil Wears Prada* is not often cited for its ability to illuminate the conditions that shape health. But there is a scene in this 2006 movie that captures an essential truth about choice. The scene occurs when the main character, an aspiring journalist named Andy, is watching her boss, the intimidating fashion editor Miranda Priestly, put together a new clothing ensemble. Faced with the choice of using one of two seemingly identical belts, Miranda hesitates, carefully considering each option. As she does so, Andy laughs at the absurdity of struggling to decide between two accessories that look, to her, exactly the same. Miranda responds:

> Oh. Okay. I see. You think this has nothing to do with you. You go to your closet and you select, I don't know, that lumpy blue sweater for instance, because you're trying to tell the world that you take yourself too seriously to care about what you put on your back. But what you don't know is that that sweater is not just blue, it's not turquoise. It's not lapis. It's actually cerulean. And you're also blithely unaware of the

fact that in 2002, Oscar de la Renta did a collection of cerulean gowns. And then I think it was Yves Saint Laurent, wasn't it, who showed cerulean military jackets? And then cerulean quickly showed up in the collections of eight different designers. And then it filtered down through the department stores and then trickled on down into some tragic Casual Corner where you, no doubt, fished it out of some clearance bin. However, that blue represents millions of dollars and countless jobs, and it's sort of comical how you think that you've made a choice that exempts you from the fashion industry when, in fact, you're wearing a sweater that was selected for you by the people in this room from a pile of stuff.[1]

Miranda's shrewd deconstruction of a very specific set of choices illustrates how our decisions are deeply influenced by structural forces, including our personal economic and cultural conditions and the high-level choices made by people with the power to shape these conditions. Andy's choice of clothes—ostensibly a personal decision, her own self-expression—is revealed to be the product of these structural forces. Her range of choice is only as wide as her context allows it to be, that which is shaped by a host of factors that are beyond her immediate control or even her awareness.

It also illuminates both the choices we make about our health and the limits of these choices. Yes, we can choose the food we eat, but our options are limited by what we can afford and by what kinds of food are available for purchase near our home. These factors, in turn, depend on the quality of our neighborhood and the size of our income, which depends on larger socioeconomic forces over which we have little control. Likewise, we can only choose to exercise if we live near parks, walkable streets, or athletic facilities, and we can only choose a person to marry from among the individuals we encounter within our community. Place, power, money, politics, and people—all the forces we discuss in this book—shape the variables that ultimately influence our health. Just as Andy was unaware of the larger forces that shaped her choice of clothes, we overlook how these structural forces influence the choices we make around health. Understanding the limits and contexts of our choices is essential; without it, we risk overestimating our capacity for creating our own health. If we think that we can simply choose to be healthy and that our health is all up to us, we will inevitably fall short.

These limits inherent to personal choice are poorly understood in public conversations about health. Our efforts to improve health—our spending, thinking, and writing about it—reflect our elevation of individual choice at the expense of nearly every other factor that matters for our well-being. Efforts like these are informed by three incorrect assumptions: that people are always able to choose freely, that all people face the same health choices, that health is attainable simply by turning away from bad habits and embracing good ones. (For evidence, look no further than the many diet books, exercise videos, and lifestyle interventions devoted to promoting healthier choices.)

We define our health as the sum of these choices, rather than as the product of the conditions that shape our world. This directs our focus towards health improvement efforts that ignore the influence of these conditions, thus leading to our continued poor health.

American obesity reflects both the injurious influences of the American environment and the ineffective nature of American attempts to improve health. Two in three American adults are classified as overweight or obese, and the obesity epidemic costs the United States an estimated $147 to $210 billion per year in healthcare spending.[2,3] An abundance of evidence links obesity to a complex set of factors, including poverty, low education, and the steady increase in restaurant portion sizes over the past 20 years;[4,5] in this sense, obesity is no different from the other health challenges discussed in this book. Yet you would not know this by looking at how the United States has addressed this health challenge. Instead of tackling the complex causes of obesity, we have focused near-exclusively on individual choice, regularly changing our diets and our exercise routines but leaving in place the conditions that gave rise to obesity in the first place.

The insistence on seeing individual choice as both the key to a healthy life and a matter of personal willpower leads to bad political policy, which worsens existing health challenges. In the preceding chapter, for example, we discussed how the legacy of Ronald Reagan shaped health. A core component of this legacy was his administration's approach to the challenge of drug addiction, which emphasized the role of personal decision-making, most famously in Nancy Reagan's "Just Say No" campaign. In a video message supporting this cause, she framed the choice over whether or not to use drugs in stark, life-or-death terms: "Say yes to your life. And when it comes to drugs and alcohol, just say no."[6]

In phrasing her message this way, Reagan promoted a common assumption: that addiction is a choice the average person is free to accept or reject. In fact, addiction is not a choice. It is, as the National Institute on Drug Abuse has acknowledged, a chronic brain disease.[7] But in spite of the fact that the United States funded the research that supports this view, the American view of addiction remains steeped in personal-choice narratives: we see it as a decision people make to flout safety in favor of repeated risk. For this reason, victims of addiction face significant stigma—a collective judgment that asks what kind of person would choose such a dangerous path. This question, of course, makes as much sense as asking why someone would "choose" to develop cancer or catch an infectious disease. Nevertheless, addiction is as likely to be attributed to the failure of people to "just say no" as it is to be linked to the true causes of this health crisis, which include socioeconomic malaise, the marketing practices of pharmaceutical companies, and the widespread availability of increasingly powerful illegal opioids.[8–10] Because we have not fully reckoned with these causes—in part because of our overemphasis on individual choice—the epidemic of addiction continues. (There is even evidence that "Just Say No"–style campaigns may make the problem worse: a 2008 study found that youths aged 9–18 who encountered advertising meant to discourage drug use actually expressed less intention to reject smoking marijuana and were likelier to doubt its potential to cause harm.[11])

Our national focus on choice has had a predictably destructive effect in the area of gun violence prevention. For years, opponents of gun safety reform have pointed to the violent choices made by individual shooters as a way to distract focus from the real driver of American gun violence: the proliferation of firearms in our society. While the narrative on guns is beginning to change, the "Guns don't kill people, people kill people" argument against reform remains an effective tactic, rooted as it is in our culture's insistence on the power of individual will to transcend the broader conditions in which we live. It is entirely true that if everyone chose to be a responsible gun owner, no one would be injured by guns. But it is simply not the world we live in. We are fallible humans, and, in populations of millions and billions, there will always be enough of us who mean to cause harm or who are sufficiently negligent with firearms that the rest of us will have no "choice" but to be injured by them. In this framing, gun safety reform is like using seatbelts to preempt injury in car accidents. It's true that if we were all perfect drivers there would be no need for seatbelts and we could choose not to wear them. But since we know that accidents will occur, wearing seatbelts is not really a choice if we wish to be healthy.

The political choices made by the people who represent us evidence a defining variable in our individual capacities for choice. The challenge for health is that the people who make these high-level choices are often unrepresentative of the people their decisions ultimately affect, which can lead to outcomes that are not always in the public interest. For example, the United States is awash in guns, perpetuating a cycle of violence, because people in positions of power made a choice to prevent reform in the interest of maximizing the profits of gun manufacturers.[12] As we have discussed elsewhere in this book, power amplifies the choices of those who have it, allowing a relatively small group of people to shape our world in profound ways. In the *Devil Wears Prada* example, Andy's clothing selection is a product of the deliberate choices of a small group of designers; Miranda Priestly rightly zeroes in on the capacity for personal choice as being defined by the prerogatives of those individuals who hold the levers of power in society (and fashion). Politicians, business leaders, and cultural influencers like celebrities all make decisions that affect the conditions that decide the choices we are able to make about our well-being. The proliferation of guns in the United States has made this tragically clear. And it means that, no matter what decisions we personally make about our health—no matter how much water we drink or steps we get in per day—we will remain exposed to the daily hazard of gun violence until a new balance of power emerges to create a new context and, with it, new options for health.

Understanding how our choices are shaped and constrained and how our existence is defined by the choice set that is present for us is essential to understanding health. In order to be healthy, we need to first ensure that this choice set is healthy. It's also what we should be advocating for—and, if necessary, agitating for—to promote health. To return to Miranda Priestly: if we want a certain palette of colors to choose from, we need to make sure Oscar de la Renta is on the same page.

U.S. history offers plenty of examples of how decisions made at the corporate and political levels typically promote an unhealthy status quo. Consider the once-prolific use of dichlorodiphenyltrichloroethane (DDT) in this country. DDT is a powerful pesticide that was used by U.S. forces during World War II to kill insects in the South Pacific as a safeguard against malaria.[13,14] When it was put to use in the civilian world, DDT was embraced by many as a kind of "miracle-chemical," praise that was amplified and promoted by both government and the agricultural industry.[15] These high-level decisions to promote DDT would have significant consequences for health. As the environmentalist Rachel Carson wrote in *Silent Spring*, her landmark 1962 book about the effects of DDT, the chemical can pose a danger to the environment and to human health, disrupting ecosystems and contaminating the food supply.[16] While Carson was not the first to express misgivings about the use of the chemical, her book showed, in great detail, how Americans were living in the midst of an unseen hazard.[17] Her findings shocked the public, catalyzing action against DDT. The chemical would eventually be banned in the United States, and Carson's work would inform the environmental movement, which, in turn, led to the creation of the Environmental Protection Agency.[16,18]

As with the proliferation of guns in the United States, the promotion of DDT at the corporate and federal levels created a space for poor health and constrained public choice against it. Unlike the problem of gun violence, though, the hazards of DDT were largely invisible, escaping widespread public notice until the publication of *Silent Spring*. It reflects how easy it can be for the effects of high-level choices to go overlooked, even where their consequences lead to extremes like poisoning our water and soil. It also speaks to the need to engage with choice where it has the greatest impact for health—not where it concerns whether or not our lunch will be a healthy one or whether we will jog three miles or four, but at the level of corporate and political policy, where outcomes determine whether our air is clean, schools are funded, and our economy fair.

Champions of personal choice—or rather, those who would rail against intrusions by government that aim to promote health—would do well to consider whether the absence of government regulation truly leaves personal choice to individuals. As an illustration, consider again the obesity epidemic. One of the most effective methods to reduce obesity is to place a tax on a core driver of this epidemic: sugary drinks. There is evidence that taxation can be a tool for discouraging unhealthy behavior: over the years, tobacco taxation has emerged as a key means of controlling the use of the substance.[19] Using tobacco taxation as a model, taxing sugary drinks could go far toward lowering consumption of these beverages and reducing obesity.[20] But this approach has not been without controversy. In 2012, New York City under Mayor Michael Bloomberg attempted to limit the size of the containers that food-service establishments could use to sell sugary drinks, drawing the ire of both the soda industry and those who viewed such limitations as paternalistic—the so-called *nanny state*.[21] Bloomberg's legislation was eventually overturned by the New York State Court of Appeals amid criticisms that the measure was a violation of individual choice.[22,23]

While it is true that reducing drink sizes means accepting regulatory limits on the amount of sugar contained in a single purchase (though, worth noting, it does nothing to curtail the *number* of drinks one can buy), the repeal of such regulation does not clear the consumer marketplace of outside interests. In other words, if the government is kept out of deciding how much soda goes into a single serving, it is not as if the decision then falls to the consumer. The right to set portion sizes is retained by the food service establishment or drink company, parties that can choose to make drink sizes as large or as small as they wish. One way or another, someone is going to choose how big our sodas are and, as a consequence, how obese we are likely to be. The choice we must make is whether or not we wish to have a say in this decision and whether we want that decision to promote health.

This is a fundamental flaw in the arguments for unfettered individual choice: it doesn't exist. In a vacuum where social circumstances or government doesn't intervene, industry will, and it's generally not for the greater good. This dynamic also applies to our broader engagement with choice in the context of health. Think what would have happened if the public had declined to push for reforms in the wake of Rachel Carson's revelations about DDT, turning instead to individual choice to solve the problem. It is not hard to imagine partisans of this approach saying, "If people do not like DDT, they can simply *choose* not to live where it is in use." Fortunately, this did not happen. People accepted that as long as DDT remained ubiquitous, a person's health options would be constrained, no matter where she chose to live. So we collectively decided to change our context, improving our ability to choose a healthy life, and the world was changed for the better. But our insistence on individual choice continues to distract focus from the real high-level choices that truly shape health. I argue that we have little choice but to change how we think about choice—to shift our focus away from individual decision-making and toward a broader view of choice and its effect on the social, economic, and environmental conditions that determine our well-being.

THIRTEEN

LUCK

"*I was so close to dying I could feel the Grim Reaper's breath on my face.*"

This is the line she uses, the young veteran, when she talks about her experience of the war. It has become a stock phrase for her. She is sick of saying it, but then she is also sick of telling the story of why it is absolutely true, why she should be dead but for some reason is not. Of course, the line is accurate, in a way. She had felt a kind of breath on her face, when the bullet jostled the air next to her cheek.

"*It was a sniper from somewhere. I don't know. I never saw him. I was lucky.*"

She always ends the story this way, with an acknowledgment of luck. People expect it. How else to explain what happened? Luck beyond luck. She knows it. It eats at her. She feels cursed now, like she used up all her good fortune in that moment on the battlefield. Ever since, she has waited for the hammer to fall, for some calamity to visit her, now that her luck is spent. While she waits, she drinks. She has a different bar for each day of the week. Today is Thursday's. The man she drinks with is an old-timer, wise-looking, who wanted to know why a young woman would swallow so much whisky so early in the day. Somehow, the veteran finds herself telling the story again. When she finishes, the old man blinks at her.

"Lucky? That was not luck. True good fortune is having five fingers on each hand, no diseases, a regular income, and managing to get through life without ever once being smashed to pieces by a hurricane. We live in a world where catastrophe hangs in the very air. To be alive and intact is to have avoided, for thousands and thousands of days, the worst of what existence can bring. You think you exhausted your luck in a split second? You are seeing it wrong. That bullet was an aberration, a flicker of bad luck in what has so far been a charmed life. Trust me. I am old enough to know."

From the day we are born until the day we die, our circumstances are deeply influenced by chance. We have no say, for example, over whether we are born into poverty or wealth, or into a country that is at peace or at war, or into a family that is loving or neglectful. And if all of these variables unfold in our favor, we must admit that we are the beneficiaries of tremendous, unearned luck.

In our more reflective moments, we may acknowledge the luck of such a life. However, we rarely think about the link between luck and health. But we should think about it, perhaps all the time. The influence of luck is perhaps never more profound than when it affects health. As the old man in the story says, momentary good luck pales in comparison to the good fortune of living a life where the conditions that surround us do not lock us into a cycle of poor health. Fortuna, the Roman goddess of chance, is often depicted as balancing on a sphere, symbolizing the shifting unsteadiness of fate.[1] In the same way, the forces described in this book are constantly in flux, poised to either improve health or undermine it, depending on the circumstances of the moment. While we can do much to shape these forces and nudge their influence in the direction of health, it remains a fact that they will always be, to some extent, beyond our control. We need to realize this and respect the role of luck, even as we do our best to fix what is in our power to improve.

In the United States, rather than accepting how chance can influence our well-being, we tend to equate health with the virtues of our personal decision-making. Good health comes, we imagine, from making good choices; poor health comes from making poor choices. In each case, our assumptions make little room for the influence of luck, of pure happenstance. Health is regarded as the upshot of doctors, medicines, and personal responsibility in the right combination, mostly removed from the realm of luck.

But even as scientific progress advances in areas like disease prevention, data remind us that there is only so much we can do in the face of simple bad luck. Consider cancer prevention, an area in which we as a society have invested tremendous resources to find ways to prevent our most feared disease. We are constantly touting new steps we can take as individuals to lower our risk of developing the disease—from changing our diet, to keeping our weight down through exercise, to avoiding environmental pollutants. But, for all this expanding knowledge, our cancer risk is still shaped by luck, and significantly so. A 2017 study of cancer genetics found that just about 29% of the cell mutations that can lead to cancer are attributable to environmental factors, 5% can be traced to heredity, and the remaining 66% are random.[2,3] These findings undercut our belief that personal choice alone is the primary driver of health.

To understand how luck shapes health, we must grapple with a paradox at the heart of Fortuna: while luck itself may be random, the distribution of luck within societies is not. Some people, by virtue of their socioeconomic advantage, are better positioned than others to reap the benefits of good luck, which translates into good health. Others are disproportionately predisposed to bad luck—and poor health—as a consequence of the conditions in which they live. I am often asked by people who attend my public speaking events: "What should I do to be healthy?" And the answer I give is: choose to be born to healthy and well-off parents. Obviously, this is tongue in cheek, but the response reflects the forces we have spoken about in this book—money, for example, and other resources—that precipitate luck. We cannot choose who we are born to, but it nevertheless plays as big a role as anything else we can do to stay healthy. There are those, for example, who are born without the advantages outlined at the start of this chapter. They are not born into favorable economic circumstances, into a stable, peaceful country, or a loving family. Other people are not only lucky enough to receive these advantages at birth, they are given even more—not just money, but wealth; not just peace, but the political influence to shape that peace; not just a loving family, but inherited status and prestige. These opportunities beget more opportunities, in the same way that having money tends to lead to having even more money, as wealth concentrates at the top of the economic ladder.[4] Under our present system, the surest way to enjoy good fortune—in both senses of the phrase—is to already have lots of it to begin with.

Why is this worth talking about? It matters because talking about it can bring about a world where luck and opportunity are more broadly accessible. While we cannot control the circumstances of our birth, we can collectively influence the distribution of opportunity in our society that informs the distribution of luck, thus increasing the odds that more might be born into the better circumstances that produce a healthy life. In other words, we are not slaves to luck. We can to some extent create our own collective luck and create a world that is likelier to generate health.

The philosophy behind efforts to create a society where luck is more broadly shared is known as *luck egalitarianism*.[5] Luck egalitarians regard luck as a social resource, similar to money or education. In their view, luck can take one of two distinct forms: "brute" luck or "option" luck. *Brute luck* is essentially another word for fate—the unexpected development over which we have no control. The old man in the story provides a classic example of brute luck: a hurricane. Extreme weather events like hurricanes can come from out of the blue. *Option luck*, on the other hand, is the circumstance, either good or bad, that arises as a consequence of our own choices. The veteran's brush with death is an example of option luck. While she could not have predicted the exact moment when an enemy combatant would fire on her, the possibility of taking such fire was something she would have known about when she joined the military. Her near-miss was therefore a predictable outcome of her own choices, her survival an outcome of option luck.

Luck egalitarians judge whether or not a social order is just by how well it distributes option luck, even as they acknowledge that brute luck will always be a "wild card" influence on our lives and health. We cannot, for example, prevent hurricanes from striking, but we can invest in the social, economic, and physical infrastructure of a given place to ensure that, if disaster does strike, the affected community will be able to bounce back quickly. We cannot control who is born rich and who is born into the ranks of the vast majority of Americans who suffer from economic insecurity, but we can do our best to create a just economic system, where all can access the resources they need to flourish. Rather than deny the existence of luck, we can make our own by creating conditions for the equitable distribution of option luck.

Confusion between brute luck and option luck can lead to misunderstandings about how we can best structure society to promote health for all. When we insist that poor health is the result of poor choices alone, we are liable to view things like disease as consequences of option luck—bad outcomes from bad choices—and fool ourselves into thinking poor health is a choice. But again: health is not a product of choice alone or even choice primarily. It is the sum of all factors—the social, economic, and environmental conditions that surround us. Taken together, these factors can shape health in the form of brute luck, influencing the lives of people who are ill-positioned to change their circumstances, who are born into a world that they did not create.

The American system of health insurance is a national acknowledgment of the ubiquity of brute luck. When we invest in healthcare, we accept that life is uncertain, that our fate is shaped by unforeseen contingencies. It is an act of humility, informed by an awareness of how forces larger than ourselves influence our health. Pursuing a system of universal healthcare builds on this awareness—which is perhaps some of the reason it has struggled to find a foothold in America. The Affordable Care Act (ACA), and its latter-day movement of Medicaid for all, constitutes a societal acknowledgment that we are all vulnerable to mischance and that an infrastructure that engages with the unavoidable benefits us all.

That the merits of universal healthcare have to date escaped America speaks to the nation's tendency to equate health with individual virtue and disease with bad decisions. It explains why opponents of the ACA were quick to suggest that the law subsidizes peoples' unwillingness to take personal responsibility for their own health. It's a belief that was well-captured in 2017 by Republican Representative Mo Brooks, who said that the

ACA raised costs for people who have "done the things to keep their bodies healthy"—suggesting that health can be reduced to proper diet and exercise and the avoidance of dangerous behavior alone.[6] This criticism would make sense if our health was nothing more than a product of the choices we make about how we take care of ourselves, if there was no possibility of random, unforeseen catastrophe disrupting our lives. But life is hazardous, and this hazard is often mediated by chance. Embracing universal healthcare is a way of acknowledging this, helping to systematize a response to the brute bad luck that will inevitably come our way sooner or later.

Pursuing universal healthcare, while important, is just a small part of righting the wrongs that foster the bad luck that leads to poor health. These conditions set the stage for permanent, intergenerational bad luck that undermines the health of millions over the course of many years. Ending this misfortune means acknowledging and addressing the structures that underlie it. For example, in the United States, black men are 13 times likelier than white men to be shot and killed with a gun[7]; this hazard parallels the danger faced by the young veteran at the start of this chapter. But while that veteran's risk of being killed by a gun resulted from the option luck inherent in her decision to join the military, black men face an equal brute bad luck just by virtue of being born in a country where racism, crime, and neighborhood risk all conspire against them. Or think about asthma, a disease driven by the interplay of social, economic, and environmental conditions that are a consequence of brute luck for the individuals who are unfortunate enough to live among conditions that cause it.

Gun violence and asthma may not seem to be related, but they share roots in the structural causes of bad luck in our society. And while these hazards may be a matter of brute luck for the people who suffer from them, they are a clear case of option luck for the rest of society. They are the tragic, predictable offshoots of our choice to let structural inequities languish. As long as we do nothing to improve these inequities, we are all implicated whenever someone's "bad luck" leads to disease or preventable harm. While we cannot control the whims of Fortuna, we can decide whether or not the sphere beneath her feet remains unsteady. That sphere is our world and the conditions that shape it. If we wish to have better luck, we must invest in improving these conditions, for the good of all.

FOURTEEN

THE MANY

It is one of the most famous sequences in movie science fiction history: the crew of the USS *Enterprise* is in mortal danger after a space battle with the villainous Khan, sworn enemy of the *Enterprise*'s commander, Admiral James T. Kirk. The fight has damaged the ship's warp drive, preventing it from escaping the blast radius of an impending explosion that Khan has primed to go off in space. Apprehending the danger, the alien Spock, Kirk's great friend, rushes to the engine room, and seals himself in with the warp drive. He heroically repairs the damage, allowing the ship to escape, though he suffers from fatal radiation exposure in the process. When Kirk finds Spock, Spock is near death, and the two friends share a final goodbye:

SPOCK: Ship . . . out of danger?

KIRK: Yes.

SPOCK: Don't grieve, Admiral. It is logical. The needs of the
many . . . outweigh . . .

KIRK: . . . the needs of the few.

SPOCK: Or the one.[1]

This moment comes from the classic 1982 film *Star Trek II: The Wrath of Khan,* one of the first movies I saw while growing up in Malta, where, at the time, relatively few American movies reached cinemas. While the events of a fictional universe may seem far removed from the conditions that shape health on earth, the world of *Star Trek* has long expressed a social consciousness that is deeply reflective upon the flaws and injustices of contemporary society. *Star Trek* promotes a vision of the future in which humanity has learned to live in peace, eliminate inequality, transcend the divisions of race and nationality, and explore the stars not for conquest, but for the sake of discovery alone.[2] It is easy to mock *Star Trek's* vision as simplistic or idealized, but it is hard to miss the core aspirational truths that creator Gene Roddenberry's vision consistently points to. Spock's dying concern for the common good reflects this optimistic vision for our collective potential—how placing the needs of the many before the needs of the few will allow well-being to flourish.

It's a useful example because it captures something fundamental about the values that create a healthy society. When Spock says that the needs of the many outweigh the needs of the

few, he is echoing a core utilitarian axiom famously expressed
by the political philosopher Jeremy Bentham: "It is the greatest
happiness of the greatest number that is the measure of right
and wrong."[3] This notion is also applicable to health, but not
in the majority-minded terms that Bentham seems to suggest.
Rather, health depends on doing the most good for the most
people (what Spock calls "the many"—and different from a
mere majority), both for its own sake and because doing so
is also the most reliable way to safeguard health for the few.
In health, there can be no health for the individual when we
neglect the health of the broader population, even when that
population lives half a world away. We saw this in the outbreak
of Zika, a disease that originated outside the United States but
eventually threatened the health of Americans. It can be easy
for us to avoid thinking about the health systems in other countries, especially when there is an ocean between us and these
seemingly distant lands. But, as diseases like Zika demonstrate,
today's increasingly connected world makes the health of the few
closely linked to the health of the many, no matter where those
many may live. Globalization has accelerated the imperatives
of promoting everyone's health. When we value our own health
over that of the group, when we feel like we can dismiss the
challenges faced by others as somehow not our problem, we
don't just condemn our neighbors to poor health; we also undermine our own ability to be well.

   This raises an important concept that is often poorly understood: in most cases, the health of individuals is not at odds

with the health of the group. Spock's heroic (fictional) death notwithstanding, in our day-to-day lives, our individual health is actually quite inextricably linked to the collective health; it is a mistake to think that we can invest only in the former at the expense of the latter. So, when it comes to how we invest in heath, prioritizing the needs of the individual over improving the conditions that generate health for all is both a fallacy and a recipe for failure. This fact has been inversely demonstrated since the Reagan administration, as gradual disinvestment in the policies and institutions that promote health have made the United States sicker and its health less secure. It speaks to a larger principle related to health and large populations, one that has been validated over time: when individuals make occasional sacrifices for the good of the group (e.g., paying into a health-advancing legislation), these sacrifices will ultimately work in the individual's favor. In other words, the best way to safeguard health for the few is to promote health for the many.

Who exactly are these "many" for whom personal sacrifices are in order? And what do these sacrifices look like? In short, the many are the statistical masses who suffer in poor health brought about by the conditions that this book is centered on—the social, economic, environmental, cultural.

The challenge here is that these vast numbers can blur into an abstraction—a mass of suffering that is simply too big for us to take in. It can make us less likely to support measures that can improve health at the level of populations and more likely to maintain our overwhelming focus on the heath of individuals (mostly ourselves and those close to us). We have examined already how enduring this focus on individual health is in our society: our preoccupation with the doctors, medicines, and lifestyle modifications that we feel will improve our health at the personal level can mean that we fail to fully internalize scenarios that threaten the health of whole populations.

As an exercise, imagine learning that your sister has developed a dependence on prescription painkillers. What would you do? It is likely that you would make every effort to help her, regardless of any cost you might incur. You would do this because you love her, because you know where addiction can lead, and because she is a fellow human being in need of help. This would be the understandable response of most able people. It is difficult to see someone floundering in front of you and not want to throw them a lifeline.

Now consider that the U.S. opioid epidemic kills thousands of people each year—roughly 64,000 people died from drug overdoses in 2016 alone.[4] While we have taken steps to address this problem, they have not been enough to stop the epidemic. Given this state of affairs, can we truly—if we are honest with ourselves—say that we have tackled this challenge at the population level with the same energy that we would apply to helping a friend or loved one who suffers from addiction?

The number of people who continue to suffer and die from addiction answers this question for us. It also hints at why we can have such difficulty attending to the needs of the many. It is not because we are callous; it is because of the way our minds work. Psychological and neurological research suggests that human cognition is a product of two fundamental systems: the experiential system and the analytic system.[5] When we witness individual suffering, such as a loved one facing addiction, the *experiential system* triggers empathy, which leads to compassion, motivating us to help the person in front of us. The *analytic mode*, on the other hand, comes into play when we think about populations—about the many. When we consider large numbers of people, the analytic mode can blunt our compassion, causing us to regard these people as mere statistics rather than as a collection of human beings. This makes it less likely that we will take action to help them. When we hear, for example, about the billions of people who live in poverty around the world, we cannot quite process it the way we can the plight of the homeless man we encounter on the street. This tendency, with its basis in neuroscience, appears to be an innate part of human nature—with which Spock, as an alien from the planet Vulcan, never had to contend.

Our tendency to empathize more easily with individuals than with populations shapes more than just what we pay attention to. It shapes how we allocate resources, and those resources in turn shape our well-being. Our identification with the individual spurs us to pour money into what we imagine will best keep her healthy—that is, doctors and medicines. The cost of this is the health of the many, which diminishes slowly through our disinvestment in improving the social, economic, and environmental forces that safeguard the health of societies.

As the United States spends more than any country in the world on health,[6] we have at the same time underinvested in the social services that actually create a foundation for health.[7] It is unsurprising, then, that in 2015, U.S. life expectancy was 79.3 years, landing it between Costa Rica and Cuba as 31st on the list of global life-expectancy rankings.[8] How is it that we spend so much to such little effect? It's because the money doesn't go to the right things. About 90% of our health spending goes to medical services like doctors and medicines, even as only about 6% of our collective health is determined by access to medical care. The other factors that generate our health include genetics (20%); social, economic, and environmental conditions (22%); healthy behaviors (37%); and the interplay of all these factors (15%). As this misallocated spending has ensured that our investment will not produce better health, it has inflated metrics on a different front: increasingly expensive medical treatments that serve to make quality care an increasingly rarified commodity. Neglecting the broader determinants of health in order to develop medicines that an increasingly small number of people can afford has led to more and more people becoming sick, even as fewer and fewer people are in a position to recover when disease strikes.

So our health remains mediocre compared to our peer countries and is, in some areas, shockingly poor for a nation as well-off as the United States. Maternal mortality, for example, has more than doubled in the United States since 1990 and is much higher than the rate in economically comparable countries: in

2013, the U.S. maternal mortality ratio was 28 deaths per 100,000 live births, while the Canadian ratio was less than half that, 11 deaths per 100,000 live births.[9] These data suggest that there is something fundamentally wrong with our current approach to health. But the fact that they are statistics—not individual stories or the lived experiences of people we know— makes it less likely that we will process their implications, that we will link the health of the many to the conditions that shape the health of the people we see each day. It is no surprise that, in the decades since the Reagan Revolution, the withdrawal of government from the initiatives that promote the health of the many have faced minimal pushback while individualized medicine has seen no limits in its investment.

Amid such rapid advancements in medical discovery, it is tempting to think that we can individualize health to the point that investing in the many isn't necessary. Yet the potential of medicine will always be limited by that fact that it works only after individuals have already been harmed or hurt by the underlying conditions that shape health. For example, in 2015, more than 10,000 people in the United States died in alcohol-related driving accidents.[10] Such accidents, which account for about 29% of all traffic-related deaths in the United States, occur regardless of how sophisticated our medicines are. And we are all at risk of accidental death, of being hit by a drunk driver, whether we ourselves drink or not. Expanding the pursuit of health so that it may do the most good for the most people requires that we address the factors that allow accidents, disease, and other preventable harms to occur in the first place, investing as much in the health of populations as we do in the health of individuals. This means focusing on the health of the many and seeing how the suffering of populations connects with broader social, economic, and environmental conditions— then investing in improving these conditions for the good of all and for our own good. This investment can range from the expansion of social services to simple changes in policy. For example, drinking fluoridated water can strengthen teeth and reduce cavities by about 25% in children and adults.[11] Expanding the number of communities that adopt fluoridated drinking water could significantly improve health. By shifting the goals from the health of one person to the health of as many people as possible, we create the conditions where all our teeth can be healthier.

To motivate this change of focus, we need a consistent reminder of how, when it comes to health, we are all in this together. In short, we need compassion. Compassion, as we discussed previously, allows us to see how our own health connects to the conditions that shape the health of everyone else. Compassion also helps us to understand how, when we are called upon to make sacrifices on behalf of the many, we also stand to improve conditions for ourselves by working toward a healthier world.

It is worth noting that, according to *Star Trek* lore, Vulcans are capable of telepathically connecting their thoughts with the consciousness of others in what is known as a "mind-meld."[12]

The mind-meld allows the hyperlogical Vulcans to gain a deeper understanding of the feelings and perspective of others; this, in turn, influences their decision-making, allowing them to choose the wisest course of action in their relations with other beings. While mind-meld is, of course, the stuff of fantasy, it operates much like the altogether real power of compassion, which can help us better understand the lives of others and how our lives link to the conditions that shape health.

It is fitting that the original *Star Trek* series ran from 1966 to 1969, overlapping with the creation of many of the laws and institutions that formed the basis for our government's once-robust engagement with the conditions that shape the health of the many.[13] These included much of the Great Society, an initiative that cast a vision of a future that was every bit as bold as the interstellar egalitarianism of *Star Trek*. As we have discussed elsewhere in this book, reforms like Medicare, civil rights legislation, improvements to our education system, and even better traffic safety laws all helped to nudge society closer to the ideal seen from the bridge of the *Enterprise*: a future where widespread equity, economic justice, and concern for the common good create a world—indeed, a universe—where everyone can access the resources necessary for achieving their full potential in good health.

FIFTEEN

The Few

"At this festive season of the year, Mr. Scrooge," said the gentleman, taking up a pen, "it is more than usually desirable that we should make some slight provision for the Poor and destitute, who suffer greatly at the present time. Many thousands are in want of common necessaries; hundreds of thousands are in want of common comforts, sir."

"Are there no prisons?" asked Scrooge.

"Plenty of prisons," said the gentleman, laying down the pen again.

"And the Union workhouses?" demanded Scrooge. "Are they still in operation?"

"They are. Still," returned the gentleman, "I wish I could say they were not."

"The Treadmill and the Poor Law are in full vigour, then?" said Scrooge.

"Both very busy, sir."

"Oh! I was afraid, from what you said at first, that something had occurred to stop them in their useful course," said Scrooge. "I'm very glad to hear it."

"Under the impression that they scarcely furnish Christian cheer of mind or body to the multitude," returned the gentleman, "a few of us are endeavouring to raise a fund to buy the Poor some meat and drink, and means of warmth. We choose this time, because it is a time, of all others, when Want is keenly felt, and Abundance rejoices. What shall I put you down for?"

"Nothing!" Scrooge replied.

"You wish to be anonymous?"

"I wish to be left alone," said Scrooge. "Since you ask me what I wish, gentlemen, that is my answer. I don't make merry myself at Christmas and I can't afford to make idle people merry. I help to support the establishments I have mentioned—they cost enough; and those who are badly off must go there."

"Many can't go there; and many would rather die."

"If they would rather die," said Scrooge, "they had better do it, and decrease the surplus population."

—*A Christmas Carol*[1]

Charles Dickens's character Ebenezer Scrooge is, in many ways, an example of how self-centered decisions get uglier as they compound. At the start of his story, he is full of hate and devoid of love. The only knowledge that seems to concern him is the knowledge of how to accumulate more money; he spends most of his time in his shadowy counting house. His sole interest in people is how they can help further his business interests. To this end, he uses his power over his employee, the hapless Bob Cratchit, to force the overworked clerk to labor in the cold because heat would require Scrooge to part with the funds for extra coal. His past, we learn, is a series of missed opportunities to be a more compassionate, humble human being.

And all of this shapes Scrooge's politics, which in turn influence health. Scrooge cares about where his tax dollars go, in particular whether they are being used to support the institutions where the socioeconomically marginalized may go to work—and make Scrooge money—until they die. (These institutions were very much a part of the Industrial Revolution, which produced both a boom in urban population growth and in social and economic challenges such as poverty and widespread worker exploitation. Dickens's depictions in *A Christmas Carol* are grounded in his dismay about how workers were exploited during this era.[2])

The political ideas that Scrooge may have supported, the type that punish rather than uplift, have not quite gone away. We hear them in contemporary arguments for scaling back investment in social services, abolishing progressive tax measures (including the Earned Income Tax Credit), and imposing work requirements on Medicaid recipients.[3] And, just as in Dickens's time, such policies today serve to "decrease the surplus population" (Scrooge's euphemism for "kill poor people") by undermining the health of the vulnerable populations who rely on the country's fraying social safety net.

While the Industrial Revolution may have created challenges for health, it also had a silver lining: it improved the social, economic, and environmental conditions of the industrializing world, improvements that included better sanitation, better nutrition, and higher living standards.[4] Taken together, these changes helped to foster health and sustain the growing population, resulting in dramatic life expectancy gains.[5] In 1841, life expectancy in England and Wales was 40 for men and 42 for women; by 1901, it had risen to 48 for men and 52 for women. However, as overall health improved, there remained those who, as a consequence of socioeconomic marginalization, did not share in the gains enjoyed by the many. They often led lives of poverty, overwork, and disease, their plight frequently overlooked by the broader society. Today, we see a resurgence of the social divides that create health divides, resulting in a large number of people whose well-being is threatened by structural forces similar to those that shaped life in the nineteenth century.

Are inequality and marginalization the inevitable side effects of progress? To Dickens, whose celebrity as a novelist overshadowed his work as an advocate for public health and the rights of workers in an era of booming industrial advancement, society had a responsibility to care for its most vulnerable members. His characters were often depictions of the marginalized few, those whose plight was overlooked amid gains by the many. This concern was a recurring theme in his works, and it is nowhere more poignantly expressed than in *A Christmas Carol* and Bob Cratchit's son, Tiny Tim.

Tiny Tim is exactly the sort of person that booming industrial societies are liable to ignore.[6] Born into a family with little money, Tiny Tim is small, sickly, and physically disabled, requiring leg braces and a crutch to move. He is, as the Ghost of Christmas Present later says, the embodiment of "the surplus population" to which Scrooge had shown such indifference.[7] But while Tiny Tim might have been marginalized by the society in which he lived, he is not marginal in the narrative of *A Christmas Carol*. Dickens makes him the emotional core of the story, the little boy's touch-and-go health reflecting the precarious position of Scrooge's own soul, giving the novella a sense of moral urgency. The story's emotional payoff occurs when, after Scrooge's change of heart, the narrator informs us in the book's closing lines that the former miser becomes "a second father" to Tiny Tim and that, as a result of Scrooge's care, the boy lived on, despite his health challenges. With this ending, Dickens gives a rousing endorsement to helping the few—"the surplus population." He argues that, even if our economy is robust, with technology propelling us into the future, we fall short if we fail to look after the most vulnerable among us.

The Industrial Revolution is long past, but we live in an age where change is no less rapid or profound than it was during the time of Dickens. Today's Digital Revolution has brought technological advances that have transformed our world just as dramatically as the development of steam and coal power transformed the 1800s. Globalization has brought the world closer together, linking fates, and health, to our shared social, economic, and environmental circumstances. The Digital Revolution has transformed how we consume information to a degree not seen since the invention of the printing press. Living standards have been raised, poverty has declined, vaccines have made inroads on eliminating major diseases, contraceptive use is on the rise, food scarcity is down, child mortality has fallen, and sanitation improvements have helped make the world a cleaner, healthier place. Just as the Industrial Revolution raised living standards, the changes of our current era have helped improve health on a global scale.[8]

But, just as was the case during the Industrial Revolution, not everyone has benefitted from this progress. Even as health has improved in the aggregate, poor health thrives all over the world, with forces of economics, war, inequality, and social stigma still preventing vast numbers of people from accessing the full range of opportunities in our age of advancement.

In the United States, we have seen how this marginalization can occur along with—and, in some cases, stem from—broader swaths of social and economic progress. Black Americans, for example, have long been excluded from their full rights as citizens. Their disadvantage is, in historical terms, a near-direct result of the institution of slavery, which supplied the United

States with much of its labor and capital in the country's early days. It was slavery, in large part, that served as the engine of America's rapid rise to global economic dominance, even while it brutally subjugated generations and created a culture of marginalization that we struggle to fully understand. The continued marginalization of black Americans serves as a reminder of how success for the many can come at the expense of the brutally treated few. Similar dynamics are at play in the plight of America's largely white working class whose continued unemployment and poor health reflect the cost of the country's diverse, deindustrialized economy.[9] Their struggle reinforces how a net positive—economic growth and the fruits of global trade—can fuel inequality and the creation of a twenty-first-century "surplus population."[10]

At the same time, we must recognize that, in contemporary America, the "few" who are most affected by these trends are actually not that few at all. Today's socioeconomic marginalization does not just affect "the poor." The term "the poor" conjures an image of people wearing rags and living on the streets. While these people certainly exist and deserve our compassion and help, a more representative image of financially struggling Americans would be of the people we see each day. The average American household of about 2.5 people takes in roughly $50,000 per year, a sum that is nowhere near conducive to financial stability for a family of that size.[11,12] For this reason, even using the phrase "the poor" can be counterproductive in discussions of the social divides that create health divides. We might instead refer to them as the "few," not because they are necessarily always the numerically small, but rather because their health is vulnerable due to the social divides we have created. Indeed, if Scrooge lived in today's world and disparaged those who lack money, he would be targeting at least 50% of the population. The marginalized few are increasingly becoming the marginalized many—or the marginalized norm. A full one-half of Americans today are lagging behind in their health compared to the top half. And the relationship between income and health today is steeper than it was even a decade ago in a country where the richest 1% of U.S. households now owns about 40% of the nation's wealth and the top 20% owns about 90%.[13,14]

Given how the Industrial Revolution and the Digital Revolution had similar impacts on the health of the few, does this mean that progress always, inevitably, brings deeper inequality and hardships for select groups? In considering this, it is worth noting the origins of a familiar word: "scapegoat."[15] The word comes from a Biblical practice in which a high priest symbolically laid the sins of a tribe on the head of a goat, then released the animal into the wilderness to wander for the rest of its days. In this symbolic sense, the goat suffers a cruel, lonely fate it does not deserve so that everyone else might live well. This practice is a helpful allegory for the marginalization we impose on the few whose fates are determined by the very forces that help safeguard the health of the many. We are, in effect, scapegoating these people, consigning them to poor health and stigma, even blaming them for their own sickness, when we need a reason to disinvest in the policies and institutions that could improve their lives.

The key difference between our modern practice of scapegoating and the practice in its original form is that our modern version doesn't just harm one goat: when we scapegoat people, we condemn them to unhealthy lives and ensure that a day will come sooner or later when their burden becomes ours. As is typically the case, large-scale health threats are felt first by the people who are most marginalized, then move on to more privileged groups.

Climate change, for example, poses a particular threat to economically disadvantaged populations, especially in South Asia, where they are likelier to live in flood-prone coastal regions.[16] This trend has been accelerated by urbanization, which has pushed poorer people closer and closer to the danger zones, even as the well-off can afford to live in more safely situated areas. This puts the economically disadvantaged in a uniquely perilous position as they are not only pushed into dangerous lands, but also as climate change continues to fuel the frequency and intensity of extreme weather events.[17] In studies that followed the 2017 Atlantic hurricanes that devastated Puerto Rico and other Caribbean islands, researchers found that islands with greater socioeconomic vulnerabilities faced greater risks of devastation as well as the subsequent long-term mental and physical health consequences from the disasters.[18] People who lack resources to escape an approaching hurricane are less likely to avoid direct exposure to the worst of the storm, which contributes to their risk of developing psychological challenges like posttraumatic stress disorder.

But just because we are not all on the front lines of climate change does not mean we are immune from this threat; in health, what goes around comes around, and climate change is an existential crisis for the entire planet. If we do not invest in the health of those who are most directly affected by it now, we risk even greater peril later on, when the entire world begins to feel what people in countries like Bangladesh, Nepal, and India are already experiencing. This means finding ways to leverage existing demographic trends, including people's increasing moves to urban areas, into the creation of safer, more resilient cities while also addressing the economic inequality that allows poverty to flourish in the midst of booming economies. As a global threat, climate change is an opportunity for us to work in concert to help vulnerable populations; the alternative, and arguably the road traveled to date, is to build walls between others' suffering and our relative comfort in the misguided belief that what happens to them is irrelevant to our own health. This belief is not only untrue; it's also dangerous—a politically born fiction that distracts us from making the preparations necessary to safeguard the long-term health of our world. When it comes to health, the fate of the few is often prologue to the fate of the many. It's been the case throughout history, whether the threat is infectious disease, violence, or a range of other threats that all begin by affecting small groups before ultimately affecting us all. Vaccines cannot stop disease unless everyone uses them; crime cannot be contained to a single block or neighborhood for long before it menaces health in the broader community. Each of these challenges punctures the illusion that the problems of the few are somehow separable from the health of the many in the long term.

Enlightened self-interest is not the only reason that we should improve conditions for the vulnerable few. It is arguably not even the main reason. After all, Scrooge does not care for Tiny Tim at the end of *A Christmas Carol* because he realizes that doing so will improve his own health or material prospects. He does it because the Ghosts of Christmas Past, Present, and Future awaken his compassion and show him how his actions link to the well-being of others. He sees how, as someone who has benefitted from the broader forces that shape society, he has the ability to help those who are less fortunate. He is also shown how arid and unfulfilling life can be when good fortune is not extended to the next person.

In 2016, my colleague George Annas and I wrote an article in the *Journal of the American Medical Association* that touched on the ethical framework for human rights (defining human rights as they are articulated by the Universal Declaration of Human Rights).[19] We wrote then, "not only do human rights include a 'right to health' for all people, they also provide a wide array of government obligations to 'respect, protect, and fulfill' the rights of people in ways that directly promote population health and advance social justice." This speaks to the heart of our obligation to care for those whose socioeconomic marginalization undermines their health. If health is indeed a human right, then depriving any person or people of health is akin to depriving them of other rights, such as liberty. In other words, it is unacceptable. Instead, the right to health must be guarded by promoting justice. (We will address justice at greater length in a future chapter.) In the present context, justice means uplifting the suffering few through actions at societal levels, particularly politics, to promote more equitable access to the resources that generate health. It's not enough to simply "level the playing field" by saying all people have a right to health; we must also acknowledge that some people are born at a disadvantage in this regard, then have the moral acuity to act on it.

SIXTEEN

THE PUBLIC GOOD

*T*here once was a park, located in the center of a bustling city. Most of the time, the park was full of people, who came grateful for the chance to look at flowers and trees for a bit instead of dull pavement and the looming height of skyscrapers. In summer, the park was full of vacationing students who descended on its grassy patches and rocky picnic spots. In fall, when the leaves changed, the wind scattered color across the hills and trails. Winter was when the park seemed most like the city around it—hard and brisk and, in a certain light, forbidding. But spring redeemed all, as new life pushed through the soil to be admired by the cheerful throngs who visited, cold weather clothes finally, decisively, abandoned.

The park was built in the 1930s by people who thought the city could use a green space where citizens might relax and exercise. It was always publicly funded, its upkeep maintained by tax revenue and donations. Throughout the *park's history, few thought twice about this. It seemed natural that something so clearly good for all should be supported by all.*

One day, a politician emerged who challenged this view. She wanted to be mayor and needed a signature issue to animate her campaign. She chose privatizing the park. She argued that paying for the space with taxpayer money placed an unfair burden on the public, who received little in return for their investment. She argued that many people never used the park, yet they were still paying for it through their taxes, and this was not fair. She maintained that it would be far better to make sure that everyone paid only if they wanted to use the park. So she proposed to divide the park into units of property that each citizen could buy a part of. Those who paid more would naturally receive the largest share of land, while those who paid less would receive less. Simple fairness.

This platform was, improbably, enough to carry the day. People began to question their collective investment in the park, wondering if it would not indeed be better to have a piece of land they could call their own. So, they elected the candidate who promised to give it to them. Once in office, she led the effort to parcel out the land. The trouble was, the park was not big enough to give everyone in the city a meaningful portion. Those who paid the most received a piece of land about the size of a welcome mat, while those who paid the least received a plot little bigger than a postage stamp. Faced with the fact that her plans had proved to be, in practice, rather silly, the mayor protested that the scheme had always been more a matter of symbolism than anything else, of standing up for individual liberty and property rights in the face of socialist encroachment.

No one could do much with such tiny patches of ground. At the same time, because the land had come at a high cost—the loss of the entire park—people were loath to let others trespass on their space, small as it was. A few tried to

forge an agreement between landowners to merge their territory for public use,
but they were only able to cobble together about two dozen properties—scarcely
enough for even a small campsite. Squabbles soon broke out among the citizens,
leading to crime and eventually a heavy police presence in the area. After about
a year of this, people gave up on the hassle of it all, and the park fell into disuse.

This story is at once absurd and familiar. It is absurd because the idea of dividing up a public park and divvying the sections among paying members would—as the fictional mayor quickly discovered—produce no benefit to anyone and would actually deny everyone the value of the park in its original form. It is familiar because the principle behind this scheme is the same principle that underlies our approach to health in the United States: public goods as a commodity. A running theme throughout this book has been how we have come to see health as something tradable or for sale, in particular in our ever-increasing spending on medicine. The underlying conceit is that spending on health will yield a commensurate return on investment, the kind we would expect from an investment in property or stocks. As reasonable as it is to wish this were the case, the consequences of this approach are very similar to what happens to the park in the story. Just as the fractioning of the park created pieces that were less valuable together than the original whole, the culture of commodifying health has made us all less healthy than we could be. And as we double down on our overwhelming investment in medical care, at the expense of the social, economic, and environmental conditions that shape health, our health remains mediocre compared to our peer countries, reflecting a state of affairs which, when seen clearly, looks truly nonsensical.

Recall Sofia. Would any pill or pills reverse the effects that a life of disadvantage had on her health? Would the best healthcare plan change the fact that she grew up with little money in an unsafe neighborhood where she was exposed to pollution? No. For Sofia to be healthy, she would have had to have access to the resources that create health, such as money, quality education, and a safer living environment. The same goes for the rest of us. Our health depends not on the drugs we buy, but on our common investment in broadening access to the resources that generate health.

Ensuring that everyone can access the resources that create a healthy world means viewing health not as a purchasable commodity, but as a public good. A *public good* is a resource that anyone can access without diminishing its availability to anyone else.[1] It can be a good, or a service, or any other shared resource that does not deplete with use. Clean air, national defense, the highway system, and public libraries are all examples of public goods. They provide benefits that are, as economists say, *non-excludable* and *non-rivalrous*. This simply means that whenever one person makes use of one of these goods, it does not mitigate or interfere with any other person's ability to do the same. If I breathe clean air, it does not mean that you cannot, just as your use of the highway does not preclude mine. It is worth noting that public goods also tend to be supported by public investment, which makes sense from the perspectives of both practicality and fairness. Collective investment helps reduce the price that any one person pays for a given public good while maintaining widespread buy-in for the resources that promote well-being in our society.

Public goods are also, by definition, the opposite of tradable private goods. *Private goods* are finite commodities to be purchased and consumed, with one person's consumption occurring at the expense of another's, thus informing the exclusivity and competition that underlie the marketplace.[2] The line between public and private goods reflects our acknowledgment that access to certain resources should not be determined by the same forces that characterize buying and selling—that some goods are worth our collective support because they benefit the whole community, enriching our lives and improving our health.

The story that begins this chapter illustrates the line between public and private goods and why it is necessary to designate certain resources as public goods, for the benefit of everyone. At the beginning of the story, the original park is a focal point for the community, strengthening ties between those who visited it throughout the year. People may have traveled to the park as individuals, but, once they arrived, they gained not just the health that comes with relaxation and exercise, but also the human connection that accompanies the use of a common space.

The mayor's privatization plan for the park marked the transition from a non-excludable resource available to all to a finite commodity. The plan was carried out in the name of advancing individual freedom, but, in practice, it meant an end to the park. More than just unfortunate, it undermined the sense of community that the park engendered, which amounts to a public loss. By turning a non-rivalrous public good into something like a market-based commodity, the plan fostered a territoriality that is inimical to cooperation and the strengthening of social ties.

Health is indeed a public good. It is foremost a resource that is non-excludable and non-rivalrous; if I am healthy, I do not in any way interfere with your ability to be healthy. The conditions that create health, the ones discussed in this book, share these characteristics. There's no health without clean air, clean water, a safe neighborhood, access to quality education, and other factors that are, by definition, public goods. And, like health, these resources are not diminished through use; when they are well maintained, their value compounds exponentially.

In the United States, we embrace public goods with varying degrees of commitment. Several of the nation's most progressive and beneficial endeavors—including the Environmental Protection Agency (EPA), civil rights laws, public schools—have faced repeated legislative assaults throughout their histories, either as leverage for short-term political gain or as part of a more sweeping shift. The intermittent assaults on these programs reveal how public goods in the United States are not tethered to a central, unified aim of promoting health; they are discrete programs subject to partisan characterizations and questions of necessity. And, as a result, like most public goods in the United States, they are diminished and vulnerable.

The United States has not settled the question of whether it regards health as a value worth upholding as a public good. In our indecision on this point, we are rather unique: other countries have embraced health as core to their national identity and count their improvements to the conditions that shape health as points of national pride. Canadians, for example, have long regarded Medicare, their country's system of universal health coverage, as among the crown jewels of their civic achievement.[3] This was expressed in a 2004 poll, when Canadians selected former Saskatchewan Premier Tommy Douglas, regarded as the father of Medicare, as the greatest Canadian of all time.

In the United States, we lack such clarity in our attitude toward health. On one hand, we very much value it or else we would not be setting records in healthcare spending. On the other hand, we are conflicted in our attitude toward universal healthcare and often ambivalent about improving the conditions that shape health—especially when this improvement seems to interfere with individual autonomy. While the story at the beginning of this chapter is fiction, the mayor's cry of "socialist encroachment" could easily have been uttered by any number of real politicians looking for a provocative slur for measures that could improve health through collective investment. Such political name-calling is just one of the many ways we have distracted ourselves from the main question we should be asking: Do we believe that health is a public good, worthy of public investment? Our failure, so far, to answer this is, in a sense, the "original sin" of the conversation about health in the United States.

American history has shown how vulnerable public good structures can be to those who would undermine them for the sake of profit or political expediency. This is done easily enough when the goal is to oppose an individual policy, like healthcare, or argue that an agency like the EPA puts unfair constraints on corporations. It is less easy to topple these institutions when we have linked the public goods to the central value of promoting health in this country. And indeed, if the public debate in the United States teaches anything, it is that it is far harder to oppose a value than a policy. Too often, the language of values has been used by those who would dismantle the structures that promote health. They have been able to do it because we have placed the cart before the horse vis-à-vis well-being, pursuing policies that improve health without first committing to health as a goal worth achieving for its own sake, as a core value and a public good. Instead, we have accepted health as an incidental benefit of disparate, untethered policies, rather than as their reason for being.

SEVENTEEN

FAIRNESS AND JUSTICE

In 2016, the sports betting app Kwiff released an ad that captured a core truth about the forces that shape our society and our health.[1] The ad features what appears to be an English pub divided into two halves by a thin, see-through wall. As people gather on both sides of the pub, they smile and wave at each other through the wall, amused at the absurdity of their surroundings as they sip their drinks and watch soccer. All of a sudden, a siren begins to wail. On one side of the wall, the sound is accompanied by the workings of a machine that propels paper money into the air, to be snatched up by the eager crowd. The crowd on the other side receives nothing; they can only watch the luckier pub-goers in downcast silence. The ad then transitions to the tagline, "Be on the right side of unfair," a reference to the app's supposed power to improve the gambling odds of its users.

Fairness is "the quality of treating people equally or in a way that is right or reasonable."[2] As most of us know, it is a quality that the world too often lacks. The Kwiff ad, while exaggerated, is an apt representation of our increasingly unequal society, where extremes of advantage and disadvantage exist side by side. The spectacle of resources cascading down on a select few while others can only watch echoes the core predicament of millions whose lives—and health—are influenced by factors like racism, stigma, and economic disadvantage. Individuals who contend with a large degree of unfairness or disadvantage (typically a product of the circumstances into which they are born and the conditions in which they live) face a lifetime of deficit compared to those who benefit from unearned advantage— the life circumstances that land some people, as the ad says, "on the right side of unfair." (This is not a binary, of course; strictly speaking, each of us is a composite of advantages and disadvantages in different proportions.) Wealth, family influence, a stable home life, a close-knit community, and the chance to pursue a quality education are all examples of the things that put people on "the right side" of an unfair world.

The societal forces that land individuals on the right or wrong side of unfair are also responsible for creating health. Poor health is often a product of unfairness, and inequalities in health reflect how the burden of unfairness can fall disproportionately on certain groups. For example, it is patently unfair that the legacy (and continued existence) of racist housing practices leaves so many African American neighborhoods in poor socioeconomic condition. It is unfair that women earn only 82% of what their male peers make, thus undermining their health by undermining their income.[3] It is unfair that climate change poses the greatest threat to populations that already suffer from the daily challenge of economic marginalization. Yet, as widespread as such unfairness is, our awareness of its power to shape our health is surprisingly limited. For example, a 2010 survey of 3,159 American adults found that just 59% of us had an awareness of the racial and ethnic disparities that affect the health of blacks and Hispanics or Latinos.[4] And while 89% of black survey respondents were aware of health disparities between black and white Americans, only 55% of whites shared this understanding. Or consider the unfairness that characterizes HIV/AIDS risk, placing blacks and Hispanics at greater danger of the disease than whites.[5,6] Just 54% of blacks were found to have an awareness of HIV/AIDS disparities between blacks and whites, and only 21% of Hispanics or Latinos had an awareness of the gap in disease risk between their group and whites.

In pursuing fairness, we are led toward an even more fundamental goal: justice. Fairness and justice are closely linked, and the two concepts are often used interchangeably. But there is a key difference in their end goals: *fairness* is the pursuit of equality within an existing social framework; *justice* considers the roots of inequality and seeks to do something about them.

A fair conclusion to the app ad would be for the people on each side of the pub's wall to receive an equal amount of money. Justice, in the context of the same ad, would be less concerned with who receives what on each side of the wall and more concerned with knocking down the wall.

The "walls" that produce poor health are the forces around us that create a world that shapes health. These are racism, sexism, homophobia, and economic inequality, all of which serve to keep people isolated, uneducated, and vulnerable. Each of these hazards reflects a form of injustice, and each is inextricably linked with health. If the world were fair, everyone would be able to access the resources they need to offset the effects of these challenges. In a just world, however, these challenges would not exist in the first place. Fairness argues for evenhandedness, an adherence to the rules of the game, whereas justice challenges us to restructure the game for the good of everyone. Creating a healthier world means creating a more just alignment of the conditions that shape health. Without the core aim of justice, we cannot effectively pursue health.

The inadequacy of fairness and the imperative of justice can be seen in the history of slavery in America. Within the larger horror of the slave system, individual slaves encountered unfairness at every turn.[7] Some would be made to work in a domestic, indoor setting, while others would be driven in the fields. Some would remain with relatives as an intact family unit, while many, many others would be divided from loved ones and sold to new owners.[8] Some would be freed upon the death of their owners, while others would remain in bondage.

Given the great spectrum of unfairness inherent in the life of a slave, it is not hard to imagine how ethically minded Americans in those days might make the case for a "fairer" way of treating slaves; advocating for such reforms could have gone a long way toward easing guilty consciences among white Americans as monstrous violations of human dignity occurred before their eyes. Thomas Jefferson once wrote, "My first wish is that the labourers may be well treated,"[9] calling slavery a "moral depravity" and demonstrating an apparent recognition of the degradation inherent in the institution.[10] At the same time, Jefferson was a slaveholder who was demonstrably unwilling to part with the financial rewards that came with owning a private workforce. He attempted to split the difference by creating a "fairer" system that limited physical punishment of his slaves and offered financial incentives to motivate certain slaves to be more efficient. But the unfairness of slave life was a product of the grave injustice of slavery itself; any such attempts at fairness were irrelevant. As long as the injustice remained, there could be no true reform, no gradual reduction of unfairness. Unfairness was merely a symptom of the larger structural ill.

This is in many ways emblematic of the role of fairness in the production of health. Some structural disadvantages are so deep and pernicious that it is impossible to avoid them when we wish to talk about health. Without dealing with the forces we talk about in this book—the forces that create a fair or unfair experience for millions—we simply cannot identify solutions that lead to better health.

It is not a coincidence that America's history of slavery is a recurring theme in a book about the drivers of good and bad health. Slavery was abolished more than 150 years ago, yet the injustice of it was so profound that it remains a core driver of the conditions of racism, stigma, and economic disadvantage that undermine health today. Injustices like slavery and its contemporary manifestations show how injustice can harm societies, and health, at the deepest level. Injustice undermines the conditions that shape health in ways big and small, often over the course of many generations. This chapter, then, is a chance to make explicit what has been until this point merely implied: there can be no health without justice. At the same time, if we do not promote justice, we also place at risk the conditions of basic fairness that require a just context in order to flourish.

While American slavery is fortunately in the past, there is no shortage of current injustices that threaten our health and the health of future generations. These injustices are recognizable by their deep structural roots and their capacity to place divides between the people they hurt most and the fortunate few they leave untouched. These injustices include climate change, economic inequality, the global marginalization of LGBT people, and the continued existence of preventable diseases that persist due to unfavorable social, economic, and environmental conditions. Just as our health conversation returns too often to talk of doctors, medicine, and lifestyle factors, this conversation has equally ignored engaging with the need to promote justice as a means of promoting health.

Justice was a popular touchstone for candidates in the 2016 U.S. presidential campaign, including emphasis placed by both Hillary Clinton and Bernie Sanders on creating a more just economy and a country that no longer marginalizes groups based on race, gender, or sexual orientation. Even Donald Trump's populist campaign messages spoke to the need to correct the structural injustices that are embedded in our economy (though he did so with considerably less emphasis on the importance of justice, save for the legal kind). The wave of progressive activism that followed Trump's election amplified calls for social and economic justice in a host of areas, including healthcare, gun safety reform, and immigration. What all this activism lacked, however, was an emphasis on the factor that unites all justice-oriented change movements: health. When we work to create a more just society by improving the social, economic, political, and environmental conditions where we live, we are ultimately working in service of better health.

Of all the activism fronts that were infused with new energy in the wake of 2016, the only one to be regularly linked to health was, not surprisingly, the push to safeguard and expand universal healthcare in the United States. This approach is too limited. Healthcare is important, but it is just one strand of the tapestry of conditions that shape health, and one that is mostly concerned with curing us once we have become sick. In this way, healthcare is more oriented toward promoting fairness than justice, and the movement for healthcare in a land of sickness is illustrative of the difference between the two. By curing us after we have become sick, healthcare helps offset the unfairness endured by those who lack access to the resources that promote health. What it does not do is correct the injustice of a system that prevents all from accessing these resources equally. It offers only a partial solution to much more fundamental problems.

True health comes from social and economic justice. It is a product of systems that create opportunities for all to live a life that is unconstrained by the forces that generate sickness. Fairness, to sustain health, must go hand in hand with justice, in the same way that pushing for quality, accessible healthcare should be combined with efforts to improve the broader, structural forces that shape well-being. Healthcare can secure the temporary absence of disease, which is not the same as health. Health comes from living in a world where no one is walled off from the conditions that allow us to be well from the day we are born until the day we die. Removing these walls means ridding ourselves of the materials from which they are made: the conditions of unfairness and injustice that lie at the heart of poor health.

EIGHTEEN

PAIN AND PLEASURE

In 2018, Gallup, Inc., released a poll listing a number of problems facing the United States, then ranking them by how much Americans worried about them.[1] Among the problems that elicited concern were "crime and violence"; "federal spending and the budget deficit"; and "the availability of guns." But the top problem, which 55% of respondents said they worried about "a great deal" and 23% said they worried about "a fair amount," was the availability and affordability of healthcare.

What this says about the American healthcare system could fill several other books. What it says about American attitudes toward health is much more interesting. In short: most Americans think of healthcare before they think of health. Americans have greater anxiety around access to medicine than around developing a disease—so much so that we are willing to place access to medicine at the center of our national conversation.

As a country that thinks about treatments before it thinks about disease, America's healthcare expenditures paint a picture of a culture that is more focused on living longer than on living well. For example, in 2014, Medicare spent much more caring for the health of people who passed away that year (more than $34,000 per person) than it did for all other Medicare recipients (about $9,000 per person).[2] As the U.S. population ages, spending on care that mostly only helps us toward the end of life has fueled our skyrocketing healthcare costs. Between 1996 and 2013, annual healthcare spending increased from $1.2 trillion to $2.1 trillion, with population aging accounting for an 11.6% increase in total healthcare spending during that time.[3] Population aging clearly necessitates us spending money to keep us healthy in our older age. But that's different from what the United States does now—spending money principally to extend life, at practically any cost.

In some respects, this spending has had an effect. The one area where American health spending produces a dramatic impact is in Americans' elder years. Whereas healthcare spending has largely failed to improve the health of most age groups in the United States, it has done much for Americans over the age of 75, who enjoy the best health in the world for their age group.[4] For a country whose Baby Boom generation is now on the threshold of their golden years, this is good thing.[5] It is not, however, sustainable or scalable across other demographics and generations. Two reasons for this: One, despite our wishful thinking, and despite our efforts to buy a longer life, we are unlikely to prolong life indefinitely. A 2016 analysis found that human longevity gains are subject to diminishing returns and generally decline after the age of 100.[6] The best available estimates suggest that there is a natural limit to human life of around 115 years.[4] Efforts to live closer to either threshold are often expensive and accompanied by losses in life quality.

Second, and more fundamentally: a long life is not the same as a healthy life. A healthy life is characterized by its richness and pleasurable experiences; a long life is characterized by a number. Is living forever what we really want?

If what we want is truly health, then the answer is no. The constitution of the World Health Organization reflects this by defining health as "a state of complete physical, mental and social wellbeing and not merely the absence of disease or infirmity."[7] In short, health is a state of total well-being, not just the avoidance of pain at all costs.

But even while the WHO defines health as more than "the absence of disease and infirmity," its phrasing illustrates how our understanding of health is largely made up of contrasts— proportions of pain and pleasure, hopefully in amounts that net a life of well-being. This yin-and-yang portrayal of health can be traced to the Greek philosopher Epicurus, founder of the system of thought known as *epicureanism*, based on pursuing pleasure and minimizing pain.[8,9] (This philosophy is not to be confused with *hedonism*, which prizes the maximization of pleasure as the greatest good.[10]) For the epicurean, pleasure was to be tempered with prudence. The ideal life would combine the avoidance of pain with the moderate, enduring joys that come with friendship, community, and other goods that can be sustained over a lifetime. The conditions that promote this type of pleasure are the conditions discussed in this book. They include education, living in a safe neighborhood, breathing clean air, a supportive social network, a comfortable income, and collective investment in the public goods that generate health. Far from the more fleeting pleasures of the hedonist, these conditions create the context for pleasure that enriches the full span of life, rather than a mere moment of it. It is worth noting that Epicurus distinguished between physical and mental pleasure and pain. According to his philosophy, physical pleasure and pain are rooted in the present, while mental pleasure and pain can link to the past, present, or future. In the epicurean view, the chief source of mental pain is fear for what the future holds. For the United States, reducing pain—and fostering the kind of pleasure that enriches life over many years—lies in reducing or eliminating this fear. Given that so much of Americans' fear for the future stems from our fear of poor health, this means creating a healthier society by improving the conditions that shape well-being—creating the conditions for epicurean pleasures and reducing pain—to live fuller lives.

In Chapter 14, we touched on the ideas of Jeremy Bentham, who argued for a utilitarian society that maximizes pleasure and minimizes pain for a majority of people. Bentham saw the pursuit of pleasure and the avoidance of pain as central to the human experience and regarded utilitarianism as a way of organizing society around this fundamental reality. As he wrote in *An Introduction to the Principles of Morals and Legislation*: "Nature has placed mankind under the governance of two sovereign masters, pain and pleasure. It is for them alone to point out what we ought to do, as well as to determine what we shall do."[11] In keeping with this philosophy, Bentham believed that the worth of a given action could be determined by how much pleasure or pain it causes. He even went so far as to devise an algorithm, the "felicific calculus," to measure the pains and pleasures of an action and, in doing so, to calculate its worth.[12] By carefully accounting for factors like the intensity of the pleasure or pain, its duration, and the number of people affected by it, Bentham proposed to "take an exact account . . . of the general tendency of any act, by which the interests of the community are affected."[11]

Latter-day thinking has brought more nuance to the work of Bentham. We now recognize that pleasure and pain are localized, subjective experiences that are difficult to quantify.[13] By attempting to measure these experiences objectively rather than individually, Bentham may have gone too far, stretching his utilitarianism into brutish impracticality or even fantasy. Nonetheless, his clear-eyed willingness to evaluate an action for its effect on the well-being of a society is worth emulating, especially as we make decisions about where we invest our resources in order to generate health.

Bentham's approach to pleasure and pain would find little value in today's placement of medicine at the center of American life. Considering how much Americans spend on healthcare, and how this spending offers us relatively little until we reach old age, a better approach would be investing in the pleasure of supportive social, economic, and environmental conditions— the things that do more to define health before age 75. This is not to dismiss the importance of cutting-edge treatments and vaccines and all the good they can do; it is simply to say that we must keep them in perspective, acknowledging that they are just one small part of the complex web of factors that shape our health.

This idea of promoting the everyday pleasure of health— epicurean pleasures rather than hedonistic ones—doesn't always win hearts and minds. Indeed, one of the fundamental challenges facing the field of public health is that it is sometimes seen as an enemy of pleasure—a stern, paternalistic entity that warns people not to pursue actions like smoking, drinking, or having risky sex lest they suffer from poor health. This characterization is only accurate if pleasure is defined solely as hedonistic indulgence. It also recalls our earlier discussion of freedom and the opinion of some that freedom should mean being able to do whatever we wish, even if it means embracing policies and behaviors that limit our health.

Just as this book makes the case for a different kind of freedom, public health informs a different, more expansive notion of pleasure, one rooted in the epicurean ideal of moderation, community, and long-term sustainability, to the end of having better health and fuller, richer lives. While limiting smoking may decrease pleasure today, it opens the door to far more pleasure tomorrow, the kind that comes from a lifetime of good health. Consider how, between 1975 and 2000, changes in smoking behavior—due, in part, to public health interventions—helped avert 795,851 deaths due to lung cancer.[14] In this sense, health, and public health in particular, is entirely about pleasure, in particular how we can maximize it throughout our lives by pursuing health and disincentivizing practices that cause pain.

Bentham's call to organize society around the principle of minimizing pain and maximizing pleasure has, to this day, a slightly radical ring to it. There is something bracing about distilling human motivation to its most essential qualities and then suggesting that we build structures around them to ensure as many people as possible can thrive. But is this not what we should be doing? Is this not how we should choose to live? The suggestion that we should dramatically alter how we approach and invest in health can seem today like a disruptive notion. But the reality is that the conditions that shape health are themselves disruptive—often negatively so. Factors like money, power, place, luck, and politics all undermine our individual rights to health, leaving us further deluded in the belief that we can control our health through the choices we make and the medicines we buy. This belief is not only a limited view of where health comes from, it is also a limited view of health itself. Health is not just how we feel after we have recovered from illness or injury; health is nothing less than everything we are able to do in life when we are well. It is building a family, pursuing hobbies and interests, the thrill of travel, time spent with friends. It is pleasure, not just the lack of pain. And sometimes it is also pain—pain suffered with the knowledge that we have a network of support that allows us to cope, to bounce back, to return to a baseline of health, supported by the conditions that generate well-being. Health is the peace of mind that comes with knowing that, no matter how the future unfolds, it will do so in a context of support.

We cannot create this context if our health spending is primarily tied to the treatments we receive at the end of our lives. To change this approach, we must first acknowledge that, despite the promise of medicine and technology, we will not live forever and shouldn't want to. We must then invest in improving the conditions that shape health throughout life; this investment must acknowledge the full range of human experience, not just the times when we are sick. It must broaden access to the core pleasures of being alive; pleasures like being well-educated, being safe in our neighborhoods, and being financially secure. These pleasures sustain us over time, so that, when we approach the end of life, we will be able to die healthy. "Dying healthy" may seem like a paradox, yet it is, in a sense, the ultimate goal of everything I have proposed in this book. Dying healthy does not mean dying at a Methuselah-like old age after we isolate ourselves from every potential hazard and, in our later years, cling to life through a series of invasive and painful treatments. It means living a life that is, yes, maybe a bit shorter, but also significantly sweeter; a life characterized by all the pleasures health can bring.

NINETEEN

DEATH

I n Act V, scene i of Shakespeare's *Hamlet*, the play's titular character comes face to face with death in an unusually literal way.
Standing in a churchyard and trading jokes with a mirthful gravedigger, Hamlet is handed a human skull. He asks who it belonged
to; the gravedigger says it is "Yorick's skull, the king's jester." The
prince is moved; he knew Yorick. In what has become an iconic
moment of theatrical tradition, Hamlet holds the skull up to his
face and laments death's power to transform even the most vivid
of personalities into nothing more than bones and dust:

> Here hung those lips that I have kissed I know not how oft.
> Where be your gibes now? your gambols? your songs? your
> flashes of merriment, that were wont to set the table on a roar?

Not one now, to mock your own grinning? quite chap-fallen?
Now get you to my lady's chamber, and tell her, let her paint an
inch thick, to this favor she must come; make her laugh at that.[1]

Despite the unique status that we now afford this scene, the
sentiments expressed by Hamlet in the graveyard would not
have struck the play's early audiences as particularly original.
Shakespeare wrote *Hamlet* near the end of the sixteenth century,
a time when no one needed any reminders about the transience
of life and the universality of death.[2] It was the time of plague,
which ravaged Shakespeare's London, caused widespread mortality, and led at least once to the closure of the city's theaters.[3]
The form of plague faced by the Elizabethans was likely caused
by *Yersinia pestis*, a bacteria that can enter the body through a
break in the skin or through exposure to the coughs and sneezes
of an infected person.[4,5] If left untreated, 60–80% of those
who are infected with the disease die, frequently within a week.[6]
These deaths can be truly horrible. As the disease progresses
through the lymphatic system, it replicates in the lymph nodes,
which can become inflamed and grow into large, black sores
called "buboes," giving the disease its name.[7] Other symptoms
include headaches, vomiting, fever, and coughing up blood.
Beginning in the 1300s, and continuing for several centuries,
millions of Europeans would die from plague.[8]

The threat of plague shaped every aspect of European society during this time, from politics to religion to art. This
was the age of the *memento mori* ("remember death") tradition

in painting and literature.[9,10] Painters working in this mode would often feature skulls and other symbols of decay in their work as reminders of the closeness of death, or they would depict an hourglass to represent the swiftness of time. These motifs would also occur in the great written works of the era, including Shakespeare's Sonnet 60, where he writes, "Like as the waves make towards the pebbled shore, / So do our minutes hasten to their end."[11] The aim of the *memento mori* tradition was to inspire humility, to warn that everything—youth, wealth, even the creative power of artistic genius—will eventually give way to death. Hamlet's grinning skull seems to say: Do not become so caught up in your own affairs that you forget that you are mortal. Death is an inescapable fact of life, and, because you will die, you must live a good, virtuous life while you can.

Hamlet's words to Yorick do more than echo the *memento mori* tradition. They suggest that the prince is startled by how quickly the living, breathing man he once knew has quickly decayed into mere remains, then unearthed and roughly handled by a gravedigger. His lines recalling Yorick's appearance and personality transition into a broader acknowledgment of death's inevitability. The line beginning "Now get you to my lady's chamber . . . " is a nod to how the makeup we apply to maintain an appearance of youth will universally give way to the grim "favor" (a Renaissance word for "appearance") of the skull.[12]

The conditions that shaped life and made death such a close companion in sixteenth-century London were, for the most part, the opposite of the conditions we understand as promoting health. The streets of Elizabethan London were filthy, often clogged with animal and human waste, and a fertile breeding ground for disease.[13] The city's poverty and growing population also increased the odds of disease and narrowed the proximity between the healthy and the sick, making the ever-present possibility of death difficult to ignore even for the most privileged members of society.[14]

Life expectancy in Shakespeare's time was about 42 years.[15] Today, life expectancy in the United Kingdom is close to 80 years, and in the United States it is close to 79 years.[16,17] The bulk of this leap in life expectancy can be attributed to the passage of the 1848 Public Health Act, which improved conditions in London and resulted in unprecedented improvements in health. Just as we today benefit from a completely different health landscape than did Shakespeare and his peers, we likewise have a different attitude toward death. Today, we think of death as something that happens to us at the end of life, not something that is linked to the conditions that shape our health while we are alive.

In earlier eras, when lives were shorter and the presence of death was more immediate, the inevitability of life's end was a core motivation for living a good life. Death was a healthy reminder of what really matters in life: family, friends, and working to create a just social order in which everyone can access the resources they require to be well. It also underscored the need to focus on factors that promote health for the broader community rather than individual self-interest alone. It is worth noting that the function of the *memento mori* tradition (also known as "vanitas," in reference to the vanity of material possession in the face of death) was not simply to frighten those who encountered it.[18] It aimed to foster an awareness of death that would inspire people to live better lives and create a better world. Hamlet's encounter in the graveyard has this effect, prompting him to reflect on how death should inform life: "If it be now, 'tis not to come; if it be not to come, it will be now; if it be not now, yet it will come: the readiness is all."[1]

In the context of health, "readiness" means creating a world where the tragedy of death is ameliorated, in part, by the equitable distribution of the forces that generate well-being in the life before it. With death omnipresent in the time of Shakespeare, there was also a constant imperative to create a better world in order to stave off death. This is, alas, just the opposite of how we approach death in our current culture, where we have done our best to sanitize it, avert our eyes from it, and indefinitely postpone it. Our investment in doctors and medicines, and our pursuit of longevity through technology and healthy living, reflect a desire to treat death like any other medical condition, one that is treatable, like measles or the flu.[19] By doing so, we have avoided tackling many of the challenges that lead to poor health. While plague is no longer the threat it once was, conditions like war, poverty, addiction, climate change, and unforeseen violence all keep the possibility of death close at hand, even as we, as a culture, regard it as something to be individually staved off.[20]

Thinking about death forces us to think about the world that we must improve in order to promote health. Two approaches to this topic are particularly helpful.

The first is the concept of "dying healthy"; that is, dying at the end of a life that has been shaped by the forces that generate health, forces that enrich life rather than just defer death. They include community, love, having a safe place to live, and having access to the economic resources necessary to maintain a decent standard of living. We should never forget that we shall indeed die, but we should all wish to die healthy. To do so, we must create a world where we can live as healthfully as possible.

Second, we should not shy away from talking about death. Death is an inevitability, as is the experience of it. Terminally ill individuals regularly say that their main priorities as they approach death include avoiding suffering, spending time with family, having access to human touch, and not being a burden.[19] Of all these priorities, only the avoidance of suffering is closely dependent on the power of drugs and treatments; the rest come from the networks of family and community support that we engage with throughout life, and those networks are built long before death becomes imminent.

Personal networks are central to our ability to die with dignity—a dignity denied to many of the people who die from the harmful conditions we have allowed to proliferate in our world. This is what "readiness" means in the context of death and dying; it is a commitment to creating a world where death motivates us to make life better for ourselves and for all as we approach a common fate.

If we don't talk about death when we talk about health, we risk undermining health in two ways. First, by ignoring death, we also ignore the conditions that often make death a more difficult or painful experience than it needs to be. If dying with dignity were a priority, it would represent a bridge to improving the lives of those who are marginalized, stigmatized, or otherwise underserved by this life. Improving conditions for the dying means strengthening the social networks that provide them support, which in turn improves them in life. Embracing death in this fashion does not mean accepting early, preventable deaths as normal; it serves to work backward against the conditions that bring it about.

Second, when we ignore death, we are also likelier to ignore the people we perceive as closest to it—older adults. Engaging with the reality of death helps us see all the ways we have allowed the world to become a difficult place for those whose proximity to the end of life has served to cut them off from the broader life of the community. The number of Americans 65 and older will more than double between now and 2060, increasing from 46 million to more than 98 million.[21] Caring for this population means creating a society where no one falls through the cracks because of their age, mobility, or disease status. This means investing in public goods like Medicare, community programs for older adults, and greater handicap accessibility in cities and towns. We all die, but there is a world of difference between feeling discarded by the community of which we were once a part and feeling valued and supported by that community even in our final moments.

Death is our common inheritance, as integral to the human experience as pleasure, pain, or love. We cannot refuse this inheritance, but we can ensure that, for future generations, it is accompanied by a better world where all can live healthy lives and die dignified, healthy deaths. The constant possibility of death makes creating this reality all the more urgent. Because we could die at any moment, we should not put off the work of building a healthier society. As Seneca wrote, "[L]et us so order our minds as if we had come to the very end. Let us postpone nothing. Let us balance life's account every day."[22]

TWENTY

Values

A central argument of this book is that Americans conflate health and health*care*: we invest almost solely in the latter at the expense of the former, ignoring the context that actually decides our health in favor of honing and procuring the cutting edge of medical science. And when we do stop thinking about the treatment of disease to think about health itself, we think mostly about our lifestyle, buoyed by the notion that if we make good decisions, we will be healthy. This has led us to emphasize individual choices about personal behavior like diet and exercise, creating the illusion that modifying these choices will be enough to improve our health, when, in reality, our lifestyle is almost entirely shaped by the social, economic, and environmental forces we discuss throughout this book. This has produced, and continues to produce, diminishing returns in the health of the world's wealthiest country.

By investing in cures for illnesses rather than improving the conditions that keep us healthy, we are now caught in a conundrum. We want to be healthy, but we have not embraced health as a value worth pursuing and protecting. And, just as importantly, we have not followed through on this value by addressing the forces that actually produce health.

It is worth noting here that healthcare and medicine, the most earnest investments that America makes in its health, are still subject to something well short of complete public buy-in. This was illustrated in the debate over the Affordable Care Act (ACA). For all the controversy it has generated, the ACA is fairly modest in its aims: it applies a market-based approach to ensuring that millions more Americans have access to healthcare. What it does not do is address the conditions that create poor health for the population it serves—the socioeconomic disadvantage that has undermined the well-being of so many in this country, from Blind Willie Johnson in the 1940s to millions of others over the intervening decades. But even the most comprehensive healthcare system would only have addressed the disease itself, not the homelessness, racism, and domestic violence that caused Johnson to live a life where poor health was inevitable. And the ACA is definitely not the most comprehensive healthcare system. Yet, even on its own, small-c conservative terms, the ACA has been vulnerable ever since it was signed into law to attacks that label it everything from government overreach to outright socialism. And yet, even if such a law had been in force during Johnson's time, even if he had not been turned away from the hospital in his hour of need, he still would have likely died of something else sooner than later; malaria was just the thing that happened to get him. His fate was sealed by the conditions around him, the conditions that shaped his health.

Decades after Blind Willie Johnson's death, our attitudes and approach to health have changed little.

Where does this reticence to address the roots of health come from? Why are we so misguided on this issue? The more I consider these questions, the more I think that, at core, this challenge comes from the fact that, in the United States, we remain ambivalent about embracing health as a collective value. Because if we are to tackle health in all we do and address all the forces that affect health, we need to value health enough to put it front and center. Our ambivalence to this is striking and curious in light of our commitments to other areas we have deemed central to our collective well-being—like, for example, our overwhelming investment in national defense.

So what does it mean to value health? What does that even look like? Embracing health as a collective value means recognizing that placing the needs of the individual above all other considerations is a recipe for continued poor health. Throughout this book, I have emphasized how our country's tradition of unfettered individualism has interfered with our pursuit of health. This tradition lies at the heart of our belief that we can buy our way out of poor health and that we therefore do not need to address the broader conditions that shape national well-being. This belief is not only wrong, it actively undermines our health.

In the goldfish example that was introduced earlier, we all share the same "water"—the visible and invisible conditions of our society, whether they're environmental or economic or other. If our water is dirty, and if we decline to invest in improving our shared conditions, poor health becomes unavoidable. Within this system, our health is interlinked. My health depends on your health, your health depends on mine. When economic disadvantage and political challenges enabled an Ebola epidemic in West Africa, it threatened health in the United States.[1] When American politics caused the United States to withdraw from the Paris Climate Accord, it threatened the health of the entire planet. When we only care about our own health, we are also likelier to tolerate the injustices that often underlie the structural challenges that create poor health for all. Embracing health as a collective value means embracing the compassion that allows us to see how the suffering of individuals connects with the larger forces that produce health.

Embracing health as a value also means engaging with the full complexity of the conditions that shape it. Forces like love, hate, pleasure, pain, place, compassion, power, politics, choice, luck, and justice may read as innocuous, but that's largely because they are all complicated, far-reaching influences that are not subject to easy models of cause and effect. When we think about health, we often ignore this complexity. We tend to regard health as a fairly straightforward proposition or as the simple state of not being sick. When illness does strike, this approach holds that returning to health is simply a matter of taking the right medications. This equation leaves little room for the broader social, economic, and environmental conditions that shape health. Medicines are important, of course, and it is self-evident that disease makes us sick. But these realities are just a small part of the web of influences and contingencies that, taken together, decide who becomes stick and who stays well. While I may think that I am going to be healthy because I run every day, I only run every day because I am lucky enough to live in a good neighborhood where there is a running path by my house and where I can breathe air that is not polluted. The air is clean because people with political power, motivated by public opinion, decided to create policies and institutions that protect the environment. At every level, a complex interplay of forces shapes the choices we are able to make about our health.

These forces also shape the emergence of disease. Cancer, for example, may cause us to become ill and die. But what causes cancer? A range of factors, including obesity, environmental pollutants, and smoking.[2] And what accounts for the proliferation of these hazards? Culture, place, industrial practices, regulatory rollback, economic disadvantage—and, especially, the interplay of these conditions. It is worth noting that the further "upstream" we get from a given health hazard, the more broadly influential and overlapping the forces that shape it become. Consider economic disadvantage. Those who cannot afford healthy food increase their risk of obesity by eating calorie-rich, nutrient-poor food, a diet of which can lead to other diseases down the road. Economic hardship also shapes smoking risk; economically disadvantaged individuals are in greater danger of smoking and suffering from its associated health hazards. At the same time, this economic status also informs our culture and the social networks of which we are a part, which reinforce influences on eating habits and our willingness to engage in risky behaviors like smoking. These overlapping conditions are far richer, more complex, and, in many ways, more elusive than the narratives of disease and medicine that we typically think of when we think of health. Addressing this complexity means promoting health in every aspect of life. It means promoting fairness and justice, making the structures of cities healthier, preventing diseases rather than just treating them, embracing compassion, fostering social connections, and cultivating the power to influence the high-level choices that shape these conditions in our society. It means engaging with all of the forces discussed in this book, not just restricting our focus to medicine alone.

I want to be clear that I am in no way against medicine. I am, after all, a doctor. I am also, at times, a patient, as are we all sometimes. Like everyone, I want to have the best possible doctor looking after me when I get sick. But I also want to live healthy for as long as possible, and I want my children to be healthy as long as possible. This book is not meant to diminish the importance of medicine or its power to cure us when we are sick. It is meant to be a clear statement that efforts to keep us healthy should take priority over treatments that are only useful once disease has already taken hold. As we discussed in the previous chapters, the goal here should be to die healthy at the end of rich, full lives, unencumbered by the limitations imposed by disease. This means taking a long view of health and working to improve conditions so that they allow us to stay well from the day we are born until the day we die.

As long as the public debate around health remains focused on doctors, treatments, and the choices we make as individuals, our health will continue to suffer and we will continue with the pattern of investment that has made American health worse than that of all its peer countries. This cycle can be disrupted by recognizing how our health has links across all levels of our lives, from the structures that surround us to our compassion as individuals to how we treat the masses and minorities of our population. In recognizing these links, a stark case is made for investment in public education, in better-designed cities, in safer roads, in cleaner air and water. In short, our beloved talk around infrastructure should be focused on creating a strong foundation on which a truly healthy society can rest. And this can only happen by including these foundational factors in our national conversation about health. This book is an attempt to do just that, to nudge the public debate toward a fuller recognition of the forces that make us healthy. I have not offered a detailed policy blueprint for how to improve these conditions, only a framework for why such polices are needed and where they might make the most difference for health. I have done so in the hope that others will build on this framework, developing strategies to improve health that are rooted in the factors that generate it. In a sense, the goal of this book is to inspire the *next* book, and the book after that, as the health conversation continues among those who want better for themselves and for their families.

The skeptical reader of this might ask: Does changing the conversation really make a difference? Does changing how we talk about something really lead to a better society and better health? History suggests that it does. Consider Lyndon B. Johnson's Great Society programs, which were part of this book's earlier conversation around power. While the Great Society had its flaws and was by no means a panacea for the problems facing the United States, its ambition and its self-conscious determination to address the social, economic, and environmental causes of suffering in this country speak well of our capacity as a society to improve the conditions that shape health. While the Great Society was conceived by the Johnson administration, many of its goals were materializations of changes in the national conversation, especially in the area of civil rights, that eventually informed federal policymaking. The civil rights movement was active for years leading up to the Great Society's programs, working to shift Americans' views on race and shining a light on the injustices of segregation. One of the key slogans of this movement was "we shall overcome," a phrase immortalized in a song that would become a civil rights anthem.[3] Often, the activists who spoke these words found themselves marginalized, even beaten and imprisoned, in their struggle to create a more just society. This violence was especially egregious on March 7, 1965, in Selma, Alabama, when protesters marching for civil rights were attacked and brutally beaten by police in an event that became known as "Bloody Sunday."[4] A week after the incident, President Johnson delivered a speech to Congress in which he said, "[I]t is not just Negroes, but really it is all of us, who must overcome the crippling legacy of bigotry and injustice. And we shall overcome."[5] This moment of powerful symbolism would inform the era's push for greater equality, as the change in conversation inspired by a social movement shaped the thinking of political leaders, and, ultimately, the thinking of the entire country, catalyzing lasting change.

In more recent years, we have continued to see how changing the conversation can nudge society in a healthier direction. In the United States, for example, the issue of gun violence has long been discussed as a matter of crime and punishment. Yet the conversation has begun to shift as we have started to regard gun violence as a public health issue. Emerging data have underscored how guns function as a kind of contagion, their presence increasing the chances of violence the same way that the presence of a disease can lead to sickness. We now know, for example, that there is a strong link between firearm access and a higher risk of being a victim of homicide or suicide.[6] Similar data have, slowly but surely, shifted the conversation from one of crime to one of health.

Our collective awareness of gun violence as a public health issue reached a milestone in a 2018 article in *The New York Times* called "How to Reduce Shootings," which advocated for a public health approach to solving the problem of gun violence.[7] The change in the conversation this signaled has, in turn, influenced policymakers, who have begun to discuss the problem in similar terms and have drawn on public health data as they craft legislation. While gun violence, as of this writing, remains a difficult and unresolved challenge in the United States, it does seem to be approaching a tipping point, one which carries a potential for meaningful change. This would not have been possible if we had not begun to talk about guns when we talk about health.

The gun violence conversation shows what is possible if we place health at the center of our policy debates. In doing so, we can then apply our desire to be healthy toward improving the broader conditions that shape health. With health as a goal, we can fight climate change, we can create a fairer economy, we can promote social justice, and we can build safer, more walkable cities and invest more broadly in public goods. And when we see how poor health is linked to the broader conditions that shape our world, we can, by addressing those conditions, create a world that is fundamentally oriented toward promoting health.

To understand what such a world could look like, let us return, one last time, to Sofia, to imagine a new story for her, one where she is supported by a society that has chosen to embrace health.

Sofia was born into a life of advantage. It was not the kind of advantage that comes from inherited wealth or privilege. In fact, Sofia's mother came from a family that struggled financially for many years. But an exceptional public education and a supportive community network had allowed her to steadily improve her situation. By the time Sofia was born, her mother had a college degree and was on solid financial footing. Sofia's birth had not been without difficulties. A case of preeclampsia had threatened her health and that of her mother. Fortunately, the country's long-established system of universal health-care meant that Sofia's mother was able to receive regular care without worrying about the cost of treatment. This not only kept her well; it also allowed her to put the money she would otherwise have needed for care toward her daughter's college fund.

Because of her stable hours working as a paralegal, Sofia's mother was able to spend time with her daughter when she was growing up. Sofia also enjoyed time with friends and would pass many evenings playing tag and hopscotch. The children's parents did not worry much about all the time their kids spent outside; the neighborhood was quite safe and well suited to childhood adventures. There were bike paths, sidewalks, and no fewer than two parks nearby, providing ample space for the kids to roam. There were also a number of well-stocked markets where nutritious fruits and vegetables were available in abundance at affordable prices due to agricultural subsidies that prioritized those foods that are most central to a healthy diet.

As Sofia grew, she was even more fortunate in her educational opportunities than her mother had been. An advanced preschool program had provided her with an early advantage, jumpstarting her later academic achievement. Her mathematical aptitude, in particular, was recognized by her teachers. They suggested that she enroll in special enrichment classes, which she did, greatly helped by the city's state-of-the-art subway system, which allowed her to travel home by herself until she was old enough to drive the car her mother bought her when she turned 16. She attended a prestigious college, then studied law and entered politics. As her career unfolded, so did her personal life, leading to marriage and the birth of her first child. At age 45, she was healthy, happy, and considering a run for Congress.

Elsewhere in this book, we examined the importance of luck in shaping health, but the happy ending of this version of Sofia's story is not the product of good fortune alone. It emerges from a world where health is truly valued, where investment in the conditions that shape health has maximized well-being for all. Through this investment, forces like the past, money, power, place, people, love and hate, compassion, fairness, and justice all help to support health and unlock our human potential. The ending of the story is significant not just because Sofia is healthy, but because Sofia, as a result of her health, is able to pursue her dreams and to expect that her daughter will be able to do the same. It falls to all of us to embrace health as a value, to create a world that is free of preventable disease and hazard, and to make it possible for the Sofias of our society to pursue their full potential so that we can all truly be well.

ACKNOWLEDGMENTS

This book would not have been possible without several people. First, this book would not have been possible without the work of Eric DelGizzo. Eric's work is felt in every page of this book. He brought to the project energy, enthusiasm, colorful anecdotes, humor, and well-chosen turns of phrase. He helped give life to academic ideas, bridging the gap between what has long lived in my mind and what can bring the reader along for the journey. Thank you. Second, this book represents a creative partnership between me, Eric, and Catherine Ettman. Catherine ably steered us as a team, reined in our more offbeat musings, and unfailingly reminded us of the story we set out to tell and of our responsibility to tell it clearly and well. Third, this book is a culmination of a long and productive relationship with Chad Zimmerman at Oxford University Press. It remains a puzzle why Chad thought this book was possible, but a happy puzzle that nourished itself, making the book a reality against substantial odds. Fourth, this book was written while I have had the privilege of serving as Dean of the Boston University School of Public Health. I am thankful to the Boston University community for supporting and encouraging my engagement in the world of ideas even as I have been engaged in leadership responsibilities. Fifth, this book tells a story about health. That story reflects nearly two decades of my engagement with academic public health and builds on everything else I have learned and written about in that time. In that respect, I owe a debt of gratitude to everyone I have ever written with, to countless peer reviewers who have provided feedback on my work, and to the readers of that work who had the generosity of spirit to engage in conversations that advanced my thinking. To all, thank you.

REFERENCES

INTRODUCTION

1. Howell E. Voyager 1: Earth's Farthest Spacecraft. Space.com Website. https://www.space.com/17688-voyager-1.html. Published February 28, 2018. Accessed May 25, 2018.
2. NASA. Music From Earth. NASA Website. https://voyager.jpl. nasa.gov/golden-record/whats-on-the-record/music/. Accessed May 25, 2018.
3. Encyclopedia Britannica. Blind Willie Johnson. https://www. britannica.com/biography/Blind-Willie-Johnson. Accessed May 25, 2018.
4. Green E. How Do You Sing Like Blind Willie Johnson? *The New Yorker*. March 5, 2016. https://www.newyorker.com/culture/culture-desk/how-do-you-sing-blind-willie-johnson. Accessed May 25, 2018.

5. Blind Willie Johnson Sleeps Among the Stars. GuitarSite.com Website. http://www.guitarsite.com/news/features/blind-willie-johnson-voyager/. Published August 21, 2013. Accessed May 25, 2018.

6. Hall M. The Soul of a Man. *Texas Monthly*. December 2010. https://www.texasmonthly.com/articles/the-soul-of-a-man/. Accessed May 25, 2018.

7. Galea S. America Spends the Most on Healthcare But Isn't the Healthiest Country. *Fortune*. May 24, 2017. http://fortune.com/2017/05/24/us-health-care-spending/. Accessed May 25, 2018.

8. Woolf SH, Aron L, eds. Panel on Understanding Cross-National Health Differences Among High-Income Countries; Committee on Population; Division of Behavioral and Social Sciences and Education; Board on Population Health and Public Health Practice; Institute of Medicine; National Research Council. *US Health in International Perspective: Shorter Lives, Poorer Health*. Washington, DC: The National Academies Press; 2013.

9. NHE Fact Sheet. CMS.gov Website. https://www.cms.gov/research-statistics-data-and-systems/statistics-trends-and-reports/nationalhealthexpenddata/nhe-fact-sheet.html. Accessed May 25, 2018.

10. Germany GDP. Trading Economics Website. https://tradingeconomics.com/germany/gdp. Accessed May 25, 2018.

11. How does health spending in the US compare to other countries? Peterson-Kaiser Health System Tracker Website. https://www.healthsystemtracker.org/chart-collection/health-spending-u-s-compare-countries/#item-start. Accessed May 25, 2018.

CHAPTER 1

1. Urahn SK, Currier E, Elliott D, Wechsler L, Wilson D, Colbert D. *Pursuing the American Dream: Economic Mobility Across Generations.* The Pew Charitable Trusts; 2012.

2. Low Birthweight. March of Dimes Website. https://www. marchofdimes.org/complications/low-birthweight.aspx. Accessed May 14, 2018.

3. Rondó PH, Ferreira RF, Nogueira F, Ribeiro MC, Lobert H, Artes R. Maternal psychological stress and distress as predictors of low birth weight, prematurity and intrauterine growth retardation. *European Journal of Clinical Nutrition.* 2003;57(2):266–72.

4. Novak NL, Geronimus AT, Martinez-Cardoso AM. Change in birth outcomes among infants born to Latina mothers after a major immigration raid. *International Journal of Epidemiology.* 2017;46(3):839–49.

5. Chen E, et al. Parents' childhood socioeconomic circumstances are associated with their children's asthma outcomes. *The Journal of Allergy and Clinical Immunology.* 2017;140(3):828–35.e2.

6. Scheidell JD, et al. Childhood traumatic experiences and the association with marijuana and cocaine use in adolescence through adulthood. *Addiction.* 2018;113(1):44–56.

7. Hingson RW, Heeren T, Winter MR. Age at drinking onset and alcohol dependence: age at onset, duration, and severity. *Archives of Pediatrics & Adolescent Medicine.* 2006;160(7):739–46.

8. National Center for Health Statistics. *Health, United States, 2011: With Special Feature on Socioeconomic Status and Health.* Hyattsville, MD: National Center for Health Statistics; 2012.

9. Krueger PM, Tran MK, Hummer RA, Chang VW. Mortality attributable to low levels of education in the United States. *PLOS One.* 2015;10(7):e0131809.

10. Institutes, Centers, and Offices. National Institutes of Health Website. https://www.nih.gov/institutes-nih. Accessed May 14, 2018.

11. Saab KR, Kendrick J, Yracheta JM, Lanaspa MA, Pollard M, Johnson RJ. New insights on the risk for cardiovascular disease in African Americans: the role of added sugars. *Journal of the American Society of Nephrology.* 2015;26(2):247–57.

12. Achenbach J. Life expectancy improves for blacks, and the racial gap is closing, CDC reports. *The Washington Post.* May 2, 2017. https://www.washingtonpost.com/news/to-your-health/wp/2017/05/02/cdc-life-expectancy-up-for-blacks-and-the-racial-gap-is-closing/?noredirect=on&utm_term=.6091a46723e8. Accessed May 14, 2018.

CHAPTER 2

1. Hamilton DW. Enrollment Act (1863) (The Conscription Act). Encyclopedia.com Website. https://www.encyclopedia.com/history/encyclopedias-almanacs-transcripts-and-maps/enrollment-act-1863-conscription-act. Accessed May 14, 2018.

2. 1863: Congress Passes Civil War Conscription Act. History Website. https://www.history.com/this-day-in-history/congress-passes-civil-war-conscription-act. Accessed May 14, 2018.

3. New York Draft Riots. History Website. https://www.history.com/topics/american-civil-war/draft-riots. Accessed May 14, 2018.

4. Golding C. Civil War 150: A Rich Man's War and a Poor Man's Fight. Ford's Theatre Website. https://www.fords.org/blog/post/civil-war-150-a-rich-mans-war-and-a-poor-mans-fight/.

5. Foner E. *Reconstruction: America's Unfinished Revolution, 1863–1877.* New York: HarperCollins; 1988.

6. Civil War Facts. American Battlefield Trust Website. https://www.battlefields.org/learn/articles/civil-war-facts. Accessed May 14, 2018.

7. Francis N, et al. The Tax Policy Briefing Book: A Citizens' Guide to the Tax System and Tax Policy. The Tax Policy Center Website. https://www.taxpolicycenter.org/briefing-book Accessed September 7, 2018.

8. Arno PS, Sohler N, Viola D, Schechter C. Bringing health and social policy together: the case of the earned income tax credit. *Journal of Public Health Policy.* 2009;30(2):198–207.

9. Wicks-Lim J, Arno PS. Improving population health by reducing poverty: New York's earned income tax credit. *SSM–Population Health.* 2017;373–81.

10. Turner C, et al. Why America's Schools Have a Money Problem. *NPR.* April 18, 2016. https://www.npr.org/2016/04/18/474256366/why-americas-schools-have-a-money-problem. Accessed May 14, 2018.

11. The Picture of Health: At Home, at Work, at Every Age, in Every Community. Urban Institute Website. http://apps.urban.org/features/picture-of-health/index.html. Accessed May 14, 2018.

12. Food Deserts. Food Empowerment Project Website. http://www.foodispower.org/food-deserts/. Accessed May 14, 2018.

13. Khazan O. Food Swamps Are the New Food Deserts. *The Atlantic.* December 28, 2017. https://www.theatlantic.com/health/archive/2017/12/food-swamps/549275/. Accessed May 14, 2018.

14. Bennett GG, McNeill LH, Wolin KY, Duncan DT, Puleo E, Emmons KM. Safe to walk? Neighborhood safety and

physical activity among public housing residents. *PLOS Medicine.* 2007;4(10):1599–606; discussion 1607.

15. Reeves RV, Kneebone E. The Intersection of Race, Place, and Multidimensional Poverty. Brookings Website. https://www. brookings.edu/research/the-intersection-of-race-place-and-multidimensional-poverty/ Accessed September 7, 2018.

16. State Health Facts: Poverty Rate by Race/Ethnicity. Kaiser Family Foundation Website. https://www.kff.org/other/state-indicator/poverty-rate-by-raceethnicity/?currentTimeframe=0 &sortModel=%7B%22colId%22:%22Location%22,%22sort% 22:%22asc%22%7D. Accessed May 14, 2018.

17. Bor J, Cohen GH, Galea S. Population health in an era of rising income inequality: USA, 1980–2015. *The Lancet.* 2017;389(10077):1475–90.

18. Trends in Family Wealth, 1989 to 2013. Congressional Budget Office Website. https://www.cbo.gov/publication/51846. Accessed May 15, 2018.

19. Inequality and Health. Inequality.org Website. http://inequality. org/facts/inequality-and-health/. Accessed May 15, 2018.

20. Income Inequality in the United States. Inequality.org Website. https://inequality.org/facts/income-inequality/. Accessed May 15, 2018.

21. Physicians for a National Health Program (PNHP). Dr. Sandro Galea on Growing Inequality. Online video clip. YouTube Website. https://www.youtube.com/watch?v=alqh5cXyZkI. Accessed May 15, 2018.

22. Williams JC, Boushey H. The Three Faces of Work-Family Conflict: The Poor, the Professionals, and the Missing Middle. Center for American Progress Website. https://www. americanprogress.org/issues/economy/reports/2010/01/

25/7194/the-three-faces-of-work-family-conflict/. Published January 25, 2010. Accessed September 7, 2018.

23. UNICEF. *The State of the World's Children 2016: A fair chance for every child*. New York: UNICEF; 2016. https://www.unicef.org/publications/files/UNICEF_SOWC_2016.pdf.

24. Sawhill IV, Rodrigue E. Wealth, Inheritance and Social Mobility. Brookings Website. https://www.brookings.edu/blog/social-mobility-memos/2015/01/30/wealth-inheritance-and-social-mobility/. Published January 30, 2015. Accessed May 15, 2018.

25. Stewart JB. A Tax Loophole for the Rich That Just Won't Die. *The New York Times*. November 9, 2017. https://www.nytimes.com/2017/11/09/business/carried-interest-tax-loophole.html. Accessed May 15, 2018.

26. Long H. The Final GOP Tax Bill Is Complete. Here's What Is in It. *The Washington Post*. December 15, 2017. https://www.washingtonpost.com/news/wonk/wp/2017/12/15/the-final-gop-tax-bill-is-complete-heres-what-is-in-it/?utm_term=.136fd21649a8. Accessed May 15, 2018.

27. About Cystic Fibrosis. Cystic Fibrosis Foundation Website. https://www.cff.org/What-is-CF/About-Cystic-Fibrosis/. Accessed May 15, 2018.

28. Stephenson AL, et al. Survival comparison of patients with cystic fibrosis in Canada and the United States: a population-based cohort study. *Annals of Internal Medicine*. 2017;166(8):537–46.

CHAPTER 3

1. Woods RB. *Prisoners of Hope: Lyndon B. Johnson, the Great Society, and the Limits of Liberalism*. New York: Basic Books; 2016.

2. Longley K. *LBJ's 1968: Power, Politics, and the Presidency in America's Year of Upheaval*. New York: Cambridge University Press; 2018.

3. Longley K. Even in the 1960s, The NRA Dominated Gun Control Debates. *The Washington Post.* October 5, 2017. https://www.washingtonpost.com/news/made-by-history/wp/2017/10/05/even-in-the-1960s-the-nra-dominated-gun-control-debates/?utm_term=.89fc91682ed9. Accessed May 15, 2018.

4. Johnson LB. "Letter to the President of the Senate and to the Speaker of the House Urging Passage of an Effective Gun Control Law." June 6, 1968. Online by Gerhard Peters and John T. Woolley. The American Presidency Project Website. http://www.presidency.ucsb.edu/ws/index.php?pid=28911. Accessed May 15, 2018.

5. Casselman B, Conlen M, Fischer-Baum R. Gun Deaths in America. *FiveThirtyEight.* https://fivethirtyeight.com/features/gun-deaths/. Accessed May 15, 2018.

6. Gun Violence by the Numbers. Everytown for Gun Safety Website. https://everytownresearch.org/gun-violence-by-the-numbers/. Accessed May 15, 2018.

7. Bakalar N. A Dire Weekly Total for the US: 25 Children Killed by Guns. *The New York Times.* June 19, 2017. https://www.nytimes.com/2017/06/19/health/guns-children-cdc-us-firearms.html?mcubz=1&mtrref=undefined&gwh=50FB6F931D9998FAC51C68D98AA9EAE2&gwt=pay. Accessed May 15, 2018.

8. Bialik C. Most Americans Agree with Obama That More Gun Buyers Should Get Background Checks. *FiveThirtyEight.* January 5, 2016. https://fivethirtyeight.com/features/most-americans-agree-with-obama-that-more-gun-buyers-should-get-background-checks/. Accessed May 15, 2018.

9. Quinnipac University. US Voters Oppose Syrian Refugees, But Not All Muslims, Quinnipiac University National Poll Finds; President Should Combat Climate Change, Voters Say 3-1.

December 23, 2015. Quinnipiac University Poll Website. https://
poll.qu.edu/national/release-detail?ReleaseID=2312. Accessed
May 15, 2018.

10. Struyk R. Here Are the Gun Control Policies That Majorities in
Both Parties Support. *CNNPolitics*. November 6, 2017. https://
www.cnn.com/2017/10/02/politics/bipartisan-gun-control-
policies-majorities/index.html. Accessed May 15, 2018.

11. steven lukes. Steven Lukes Website. https://stevenlukes.net/.
Accessed May 15, 2018.

12. Swartz DL. Recasting power in its third dimension. *Theory and
Society*. 2007;36(1):103–9.

13. Siegel KR, et al. Association of higher consumption of
foods derived from subsidized commodities with adverse
cardiometabolic risk among US adults. *JAMA Internal Medicine*.
2016;176(8):1124–32.

14. Milbank D. Vice President Biden's Gay-Marriage Gaffe Is Mess
for White House. *The Washington Post*. May 7, 2012. https://www.
washingtonpost.com/opinions/2012/05/07/gIQAOzFw8T_
story.html?utm_term=.115ef838bd89. Accessed May 15, 2018.

15. Berman T. Joe Biden's *Will & Grace* Shout-out Was "One of the
Proudest Moments" of Debra Messing's Life. *New York Magazine*.
May 10, 2012. http://nymag.com/daily/intelligencer/2012/05/
debra-messing-biden-gay-marriage-will-grace.html. Accessed
May 15, 2018.

16. Caro RA. LBJ Goes for Broke. *Smithsonian*. June 2002. https://
www.smithsonianmag.com/history/lbj-goes-for-broke-
64104277/. Accessed May 15, 2018.

17. History. 1965: Johnson Signs Medicare into Law. History Website.
https://www.history.com/this-day-in-history/johnson-signs-
medicare-into-law. Accessed May 15, 2018.

18. Zelizer JE. How Medicare Was Made. *The New Yorker*. February 15, 2015. https://www.newyorker.com/news/news-desk/medicare-made. Accessed May 15, 2018.

19. Rose S. *Financing Medicaid: Federalism and the Growth of America's Health Care Safety Net*. Ann Arbor: University of Michigan Press; 2013.

20. Bloch M, Fairfield H, Harris J, Keller J, Willis D, Bennett K. How the NRA Rates Lawmakers. *The New York Times*. https://archive. nytimes.com/www.nytimes.com/interactive/2012/12/19/us/ politics/nra.html. Updated December 19, 2012. Accessed May 16, 2018.

21. Jamieson C. Gun Violence Research: History of the Federal Funding Freeze. *Psychological Science Agenda*. February 2013. http:// www.apa.org/science/about/psa/2013/02/gun-violence.aspx. Accessed May 16, 2018.

22. Achenbach J, Higham S, Horwitz S. How NRA's True Believers Converted a Marksmanship Group into a Mighty Gun Lobby. *The Washington Post*. January 12, 2013. https://www.washingtonpost.com/ politics/how-nras-true-believers-converted-a-marksmanship-group-into-a-mighty-gun-lobby/2013/01/12/51c62288-59b9-11e2-88d0-c4cf65c3ad15_story.html?utm_term=.25d629cb6dde. Accessed May 16, 2018.

23. Viral Hepatitis and Men Who Have Sex with Men. Centers for Disease Control and Prevention Website. https://www.cdc. gov/hepatitis/Populations/MSM.htm. Updated May 16, 2018. Accessed May 16, 2018.

24. Substance Use and SUDs in LGBT Populations. National Institute on Drug Abuse Website. https://www.drugabuse.gov/ related-topics/substance-use-suds-in-lgbt-populations.Updated September 2017. Accessed May 16, 2018.

25. Case P, et al. Sexual orientation, health risk factors, and physical functioning in the Nurses' Health Study II. *Journal of Women's Health.* 2004;13(9):1033–47.

26. Clements-Nolle K, Marx R, Katz M. Attempted suicide among transgender persons: the influence of gender-based discrimination and victimization. *Journal of Homosexuality.* 2006;51(3):53–69.

27. Time's Up Now Website. https://www.timesupnow.com/. Accessed May 16, 2018.

28. Centers for Disease Control and Prevention. Achievements in Public Health, 1900–1999: tobacco use. *Morbidity and Mortality Weekly Report (MMWR).* 1999;48(43):986–93.

29. Smoking & Cardiovascular Disease (Heart Disease). American Heart Association Website. http://www.heart.org/HEARTORG/HealthyLiving/QuitSmoking/QuittingResources/Smoking-Cardiovascular-Disease_UCM_305187_Article.jsp#.WvyBmdMvzVo. Updated February 17, 2014. Accessed May 16, 2018.

30. McGreal C. Robert Caro: A Life with LBJ and the Pursuit of Power. *The Guardian.* June 9, 2012. https://www.theguardian.com/world/2012/jun/10/lyndon-b-johnson-robert-caro-biography. Accessed May 16, 2018.

CHAPTER 4

1. Aristotle, trans. by Benjamin Jowett. *The Complete Works of Aristotle: The Revised Oxford Translation,* ed. by Jonathan Barnes. Princeton, NJ: Princeton University Press; 1984.

2. Yemen Crisis: Who Is Fighting Whom? *BBC News.* January 30, 2018. http://www.bbc.com/news/world-middle-east-29319423. Accessed May 16, 2018.

3. How to Lose a Drug War: Heroin, HIV, and the Russian Federation. Pulitzer Center Website. https://pulitzercenter.org/project/russia-hiv-aids-heroin-drug-abuse-intervention-youth. Accessed May 16, 2018.

4. Burton TI. How Russia's Strongmen Use Homophobia to Stay in Power. *Vox.* August 2, 2017. https://www.vox.com/identities/2017/8/2/16034630/russias-strongmen-homophobia-power-kadyrov-chechnya-lgbtq. Accessed May 16, 2018.

5. HIV and AIDS in Russia. Avert Website. https://www.avert.org/professionals/hiv-around-world/eastern-europe-central-asia/russia. Accessed May 16, 2018.

6. Brock R. *Greek Political Imagery: From Homer to Aristotle.* London: Bloomsbury; 2013.

7. Isaacs J. The Ten Plagues. Chabad.org Website. https://www.chabad.org/library/article_cdo/aid/1653/jewish/The-Ten-Plagues.htm. Accessed May 16, 2018.

8. Bor J. Diverging life expectancies and voting patterns in the 2016 US presidential election. *American Journal of Public Health.* 2017;107(10):1560–62.

9. Centers for Disease Control and Prevention. Ten great public health achievements—United States, 1900–1990. *Morbidity and Mortality Weekly Report (MMWR).* 1999;48(12):241–43.

10. Centers for Disease Control and Prevention. Achievements in public health, 1900–1999: motor-vehicle safety. *Morbidity and Mortality Weekly Report (MMWR).* 1999;48(18):369–74.

11. Olmstead T. Highway Safety Act of 1966. Encyclopedia.com Website. https://www.encyclopedia.com/history/encyclopedias-almanacs-transcripts-and-maps/highway-safety-act-1966. Accessed May 16, 2018.

12. Intervention Fact Sheets: Primary Enforcement of Seat Belt Laws. Centers for Disease Control and Prevention Website. https://www.cdc.gov/motorvehiclesafety/calculator/factsheet/seatbelt.html. Updated December 2, 2015. Accessed May 16, 2018.

13. Global Road Safety Partnership Website. https://www.grsproadsafety.org/. Accessed May 16, 2018.

14. National Highway Traffic Safety Administration Website. https://www.nhtsa.gov/. Accessed May 16, 2018.

15. National Transportation Safety Board Website. https://www.ntsb.gov/Pages/default.aspx. Accessed May 16, 2018.

16. Galea S. Climate Change Is Making Us Sick. *Cognoscenti*. June 2, 2017. http://www.wbur.org/cognoscenti/2017/06/02/climate-change-is-making-us-sick. Accessed May 16, 2018.

17. Fink DS, Galea S. Life course epidemiology of trauma and related psychopathology in civilian populations. *Current Psychiatry Reports*. 2015;17(5):31.

18. Climate Change and Disasters. UNHCR—The UN Refugee Agency Website. http://www.unhcr.org/en-us/climate-change-and-disasters.html. Accessed May 16, 2018.

19. Gushulak B, Weekers J, Macpherson D. Migrants and emerging public health issues in a globalized world: threats, risks and challenges, an evidence-based framework. *Emerging Health Threats Journal*. 2009;2:e10.

20. Andrees B, Belser P, eds. *Forced Labor: Coercion and Exploitation in the Private Economy*. Boulder, CO: Lynne Rienner Publishers; 2009.

21. Coffel ED, Horton RM, de Sherbinin A. Temperature and humidity based projections of a rapid rise in global heat stress exposure during the 21st century. *Environmental Research Letters*. 2017;13(1):014001.

22. Facts: Climate Change: How Do We Know? NASA: Climate Change and Global Warming Website. https://climate.nasa.gov/evidence/. Accessed May 17, 2018.

23. Davey M. Humans Causing Climate to Change 170 Times Faster Than Natural Forces. *The Guardian*. February 12, 2017. https://www.theguardian.com/environment/2017/feb/12/humans-causing-climate-to-change-170-times-faster-than-natural-forces. Accessed May 17, 2018.

24. Lee A. Moving the Overton Window. *Big Think*. http://bigthink.com/daylight-atheism/moving-the-overton-window. Accessed May 17, 2018.

25. Tanenhaus S. The Architect of the Radical Right. *The Atlantic*. July/August 2017 issue. https://www.theatlantic.com/magazine/archive/2017/07/the-architect-of-the-radical-right/528672/. Accessed May 17, 2018.

26. Rothman L. Here's Why the Environmental Protection Agency Was Created. *TIME*. March 22, 2017. http://time.com/4696104/environmental-protection-agency-1970-history/. Accessed May 17, 2018.

27. Nixon R. "Annual Message to the Congress on the State of the Union." January 22, 1970. Online by Gerhard Peters and John T. Woolley. The American Presidency Project Website. http://www.presidency.ucsb.edu/ws/?pid=2921. Accessed May 17, 2018.

28. Carswell C. How Reagan's EPA Chief Paved the Way for Trump's Assault on the Agency. *The New Republic*. March 21, 2017. https://newrepublic.com/article/141471/reagans-epa-chief-paved-way-trumps-assault-agency. Accessed May 17, 2018.

29. Reagan R. "Inaugural Address." January 20, 1981. Online by Gerhard Peters and John T. Woolley. The American Presidency

Project Website. http://www.presidency.ucsb.edu/ws/ ?pid=43130. Accessed May 17, 2018.

30. Sellers C. Trump and Pruitt Are the Biggest Threat to the EPA in Its 47 Years of Existence. *Vox.* July 1, 2017. https://www.vox.com/2017/7/1/15886420/pruitt-threat-epa. Accessed May 17, 2018.

31. Ouroboros. Encyclopedia Britannica Website. https://www.britannica.com/topic/Ouroboros. Accessed May 17, 2018.

32. James Madison, *Federalist* 10, in Hamilton A, Madison J, Jay J. *The Federalist,* ed. by Jacob E. Cooke. Middletown, CT: Wesleyan University Press; 1961.

33. Taylor R, Rieger A. Medicine as social science: Rudolf Virchow on the typhus epidemic in Upper Silesia. *International Journal of Health Services.* 1985;15(4):547–59.

34. Azar HA. Rudolf Virchow, not just a pathologist: a re-examination of the report on the typhus epidemic in Upper Silesia. *Annals of Diagnostic Pathology.* 1997;1(1):65–71.

35. Drotman DP. Emerging infectious diseases: a brief biographical heritage. *Emerging Infectious Diseases.* 1998;4(3):372–73.

36. The Universal Declaration of Human Rights. The United Nations Website. http://www.un.org/en/universal-declaration-human-rights/. Accessed May 17, 2018.

CHAPTER 5

1. Centers for Disease Control and Prevention. *Asthma Facts—CDC's National Asthma Control Program Grantees.* Atlanta, GA: Department of Health and Human Services, Centers for Disease Control and Prevention; 2013.

2. Gern JE. The urban environment and childhood asthma study. *Journal of Allergy and Clinical Immunology.* 2010;125(3):545–49.

3. Ramey C. America's Unfair Rules of the Road. *Slate.* February 27, 2015. http://www.slate.com/articles/news_and_politics/politics/2015/02/america_s_transportation_system_discriminates_against_minorities_and_poor.html. Accessed May 18, 2018.

4. Pénard-Morand C, et al. Long-term exposure to close-proximity air pollution and asthma and allergies in urban children. *European Respiratory Journal.* 2010;36(1):33–40.

5. Khreis H, Nieuwenhuijsen MJ. Traffic-related air pollution and childhood asthma: recent advances and remaining gaps in the exposure assessment methods. *International Journal of Environmental Research and Public Health.* 2017;14(3):pii:E312.

6. Wallace DF. "Plain Old Untrendy Troubles and Emotions." *The Guardian.* September 19, 2008. https://www.theguardian.com/books/2008/sep/20/fiction. Accessed May 18, 2018.

7. Galea S, Vlahov D. Urban health: evidence, challenges, and directions. *Annual Review of Public Health.* 2005;26:341–65.

8. Weich S, Blanchard M, Prince M, Burton E, Erens B, Sproston K. Mental health and the built environment: cross-sectional survey of individual and contextual risk factors for depression. *British Journal of Psychiatry.* 2002;180:428–33.

9. O'Sullivan F. Did London's Housing Crisis Help Spark a Fatal Blaze? *CityLab.* June 14, 2017. https://www.citylab.com/equity/2017/06/grenfell-tower-fire/530262/. Accessed May 18, 2018.

10. BBC News. Grenfell Tower Final Death Toll Stands at 71. *BBC News.* November 16, 2017. http://www.bbc.com/news/uk-42008279. Accessed May 18, 2018.

11. Veitch J, Abbott G, Kaczynski AT, Wilhelm Stanis SA, Besenyi GM, Lamb KE. Park availability and physical activity, TV time, and overweight and obesity among women: findings from Australia and the United States. *Health & Place.* 2016;38:96–102.

12. Astell-Burt T, Mitchell R, Hartig T. The association between green space and mental health varies across the lifecourse. A longitudinal study. *Journal of Epidemiology and Community Health.* 2014;68(6):578–83.

13. Barnett E, Casper M. A definition of "social environment." *American Journal of Public Health.* 2001;91(3):465.

14. Faris REL, Dunham HW. *Mental Disorders in Urban Areas: An Ecological Study of Schizophrenia and Other Psychoses.* Chicago, IL: Chicago University Press; 1939.

15. Christensen J. PTSD from Your ZIP Code: Urban Violence and the Brain. *CNN.* March 27, 2015. https://www.cnn.com/2014/03/27/health/urban-ptsd-problems/. Accessed May 19, 2018.

16. Ahern J, Galea S, Hubbard A, Syme LS. Neighborhood smoking norms modify the relation between collective efficacy and smoking behavior. *Drug and Alcohol Dependence.* 2009;100(1–2):138–45.

17. Suglia SF, Shelton RC, Hsiao A, Wang YC, Rundle A, Link BG. Why the neighborhood social environment is critical in obesity prevention. *Journal of Urban Health.* 2016;93(1):206–12.

18. Spencer N, Logan S. Social influences on birth weight. *Journal of Epidemiology & Community Health.* 2002;56(5):326–27.

19. Social capital. Dictionary.com Website. http://www.dictionary.com/browse/social-capital. Accessed May 19, 2018.

20. Aldrich DP, Meyer MA. Social capital and community resilience. *American Behavioral Scientist.* 2015;59(2):254–69.

21. Asthma Treatments. WebMD Website. https://www.webmd.com/asthma/guide/asthma-treatments#1. Accessed May 19, 2018.

22. Alexander D, Currie J. Is it who you are or where you live? Residential segregation and racial gaps in childhood asthma. *Journal of Health Economics.* 2017;55:186–200.

23. Dowell JA. Social interactions and children with asthma. *Journal of Child Health Care.* 2016;20(4):512–20.

24. Wilmot NA, Dauner KN. Examination of the influence of social capital on depression in fragile families. *Journal of Epidemiology & Community Health.* 2017;71(3):296–302.

25. HUD Issues Final Rule to Help Children Exposed to Lead Paint Hazards. US Department of Housing and Urban Development Website. https://www.hud.gov/press/press_releases_media_advisories/2017/HUDNo_17-006.Released January 13, 2017. Accessed May 19, 2018.

26. Bouchard M, et al. Blood lead levels and major depressive disorder, panic disorder, and generalized anxiety disorder in US young adults. *Archives of General Psychiatry.* 2009;66(12):1313–19.

27. Flora G, Gupta D, Tiwari A. Toxicity of lead: a review with recent updates. *Interdisciplinary Toxicology.* 2012;5(2):47–58.

28. World's Population Increasingly Urban with More Than Half Living in Urban Areas. United Nations Website. http://www.un.org/en/development/desa/news/population/world-urbanization-prospects-2014.html. Published July 10, 2014. Accessed May 19, 2018.

CHAPTER 6

1. Sartre J-P, trans. by Gilbert S, Abel L. *No Exit, and Three Other Plays.* New York: Vintage Books; 1955.

2. Pennisi E. How Humans Became Social. *Wired.* November 9, 2011. https://www.wired.com/2011/11/humans-social/. Accessed May 19, 2018.

3. Donne J. Devotions upon Emergent Occasions: Meditation XVII. Christian Classics Ethereal Library Website. http://www.ccel.org/ccel/donne/devotions.txt. Accessed May 19, 2018.

4. Umberson D, Montez JK. Social relationships and health: a flashpoint for health policy. *Journal of Health and Social Behavior.* 2010;51(Suppl):S54–S66.

5. Yang YC, Boen C, Gerken K, Li T, Schorpp K, Harris KM. Social relationships and physiological determinants of longevity across the human life span. *Proceedings of the National Academy of Sciences of the United States of America.* 2016;113(3):578–83.

6. Vaccines Protect Your Community. Vaccines.gov Website. https://www.vaccines.gov/basics/work/protection/index.html. Accessed May 19, 2018.

7. Phadke VK, Bednarczyk RA, Salmon DA, Omer SB. Association between vaccine refusal and vaccine-preventable diseases in the United States: a review of measles and pertussis. *JAMA: The Journal of the American Medical Association.* 2016;315(11):1149–58.

8. Kolata G. Obesity spreads to friends, study concludes. *The New York Times.* July 25, 2007. https://www.nytimes.com/2007/07/25/health/25iht-fat.4.6830240.html?mtrref=undefined. Accessed May 19, 2018.

9. Christakis NA, Fowler JH. The spread of obesity in a large social network over 32 years. *The New England Journal of Medicine.* 2007;357(4):370–79.

10. Freudenberg N, Galea S, Vlahov D, eds. *Cities and the Health of the Public.* Nashville, TN: Vanderbilt University Press; 2006.

11. Social contagion. Oxford Reference Website. http://www.oxfordreference.com/view/10.1093/acref/9780199534067.001.0001/acref-9780199534067-e-7741. Accessed May 20, 2018.

12. Social Learning Theory (Bandura). Learning Theories and Models Summaries Website. https://www.learning-theories.

com/social-learning-theory-bandura.html. Accessed May 20, 2018.

13. Christakis NA, Fowler JH. The collective dynamics of smoking in a large social network. *The New England Journal of Medicine.* 2008;358(21):2249–58.

14. JN Rosenquist, JH Fowler, NA Christakis. Social network determinants of depression. *Molecular Psychiatry.* 2011;16(3):273–81.

15. Mednick SC, Christakis NA, Fowler JH. The spread of sleep loss influences drug use in adolescent social networks. *PLOS One.* 2010;5(3):e9775.

16. Datar A, Nicosia N. Assessing social contagion in body mass index, overweight, and obesity using a natural experiment. *JAMA Pediatrics.* 2018;172(3):239–46.

17. Mesic A. POV: Solitary Confinement Offends Basic Humanity. *BU Today.* February 6, 2018. http://www.bu.edu/today/2018/ pov-solitary-confinement-offends-basic-humanity/ ?utm_source=social&utm_medium=TWITTER&utm_ campaign=prbuexperts. Accessed May 20, 2018.

18. Holt-Lunstad J, Smith TB, Baker M, Harris T, Stephenson D. Loneliness and social isolation as risk factors for mortality: a meta-analytic review. *Perspectives on Psychological Science.* 2015;10(2):227–37.

19. Holt-Lunstad J, Smith TB, Layton JB. Social relationships and mortality risk: a meta-analytic review. *PLOS Medicine.* 2010;7(7):e1000316.

20. Yeginsu C. UK Appoints a Minister for Loneliness. *The New York Times.* January 17, 2018. https://www.nytimes.com/2018/01/ 17/world/europe/uk-britain-loneliness.html. Accessed May 20, 2018.

21. The Beatles. Eleanor Rigby Lyrics. LyricsFreak.com Website. http://www.lyricsfreak.com/b/beatles/eleanor+rigby_ 10026674.html. Accessed May 20, 2018.

22. Definition of Addiction. American Society of Addiction Medicine Website. https://www.asam.org/resources/definition-of-addiction. Accessed May 20, 2018.

23. Hobbes M. Together Alone: The Epidemic of Gay Loneliness. *Huffington Post Highline.* March 2, 2017. https://highline. huffingtonpost.com/articles/en/gay-loneliness/. Accessed May 20, 2018.

24. Olien J. Loneliness Is Deadly. *Slate.* August 23, 2013. http://www. slate.com/articles/health_and_science/medical_examiner/ 2013/08/dangers_of_loneliness_social_isolation_is_deadlier_ than_obesity.html. Accessed May 20, 2018.

25. Burholt V, Windle G, Morgan DJ, on behalf of the CFAS Wales team. A social model of loneliness: the roles of disability, social resources, and cognitive impairment. *The Gerontologist.* 2017;57(6):1020–30.

26. Loneliness Among Older Adults. AARP.org Website. https://www. aarp.org/content/dam/aarp/research/surveys_statistics/general/2012/loneliness-fact-sheet.doi.10.26419%252Fres.00064.002. pdf. Accessed May 20, 2018.

27. van den Broek T. Gender differences in the correlates of loneliness among Japanese persons aged 50–70. *Australasian Journal on Ageing.* 2017;36(3):234–37.

28. Perissinotto CM, Stijacic Cenzer I, Covinsky KE. Loneliness in older persons: a predictor of functional decline and death. *Archives of Internal Medicine.* 2012;172(14):1078–83.

29. Gale CR, Westbury L, Cooper C. Social isolation and loneliness as risk factors for the progression of frailty: the English Longitudinal Study of Ageing. *Age and Ageing.* 2018;47(3):392–97.

30. Tan Chen V. All Hollowed Out. *The Atlantic.* January 16, 2016. https://www.theatlantic.com/business/archive/2016/01/white-working-class-poverty/424341/. Accessed May 20, 2018.

31. Case A, Deaton A. Rising morbidity and mortality in mid-life among white non-Hispanic Americans in the 21st century. *Proceedings of the National Academy of Sciences of the United States of America.* 2015;112(49):15078–83.

32. Case A, Deaton A. Mortality and Morbidity in the 21st Century. Brookings Website. https://www.brookings.edu/bpea-articles/mortality-and-morbidity-in-the-21st-century/. Published March 23, 2017. Accessed May 20, 2018.

33. Lawson A. Home Owners' Loan Corporation. Encyclopedia.com Website. https://www.encyclopedia.com/history/united-states-and-canada/us-history/home-owners-loan-corporation. Accessed May 20, 2018.

34. Hunt DB. Redlining. Encyclopedia of Chicago Website. http://www.encyclopedia.chicagohistory.org/pages/1050.html. Accessed May 20, 2018.

35. DeParle J. When Government Drew the Color Line. *The New York Review of Books.* February 22, 2018. http://www.nybooks.com/articles/2018/02/22/when-government-drew-the-color-line/. Accessed May 20, 2018.

36. Eligon J, Gebeloff R. Affluent and Black, and Still Trapped by Segregation. *The New York Times.* August 20, 2016. https://www.nytimes.com/2016/08/21/us/milwaukee-segregation-wealthy-black-families.html. Accessed May 20, 2018.

37. Social Explorer Featured in NY Times Article on Segregation of Affluent Black Families. Social Explorer Website. https://www.socialexplorer.com/blog/post/social-explorer-featured-in-ny-times-article-on-segregation-of-affluent-black-families-5645. Accessed May 20, 2018.

38. Sullivan A. The Poison We Pick. *New York* Magazine. February 20, 2018. http://nymag.com/daily/intelligencer/2018/02/americas-opioid-epidemic.html. Accessed May 20, 2018.

39. Health Is Other People. Kamwell Website. http://kamwell.com/health-is-other-people/. Accessed May 20, 2018.

CHAPTER 7

1. McCall Smith A. WH Auden Can Teach Us Not to Be Afraid. *The New Republic*. September 20, 2013. https://newrepublic.com/article/114792/w-h-auden-can-teach-us-not-be-afraid. Accessed May 20, 2018.

2. Auden WH. *September 1, 1939*. Academy of American Poets Website. From *Another Time*, by WH Auden. Random House; 1940. https://www.poets.org/poetsorg/poem/september-1-1939. Accessed May 20, 2018.

3. 1939: Germans Invade Poland. History Website. https://www.history.com/this-day-in-history/germans-invade-poland. Accessed May 20, 2018.

4. Auden WH. *Epitaph on a Tyrant*. Academy of American Poets Website. From *Another Time*, by WH Auden. Random House; 1940. https://www.poets.org/poetsorg/poem/epitaph-tyrant. Accessed May 20, 2018.

5. Hitchens C. The Verbal Revolution. *Slate*. August 25, 2008. http://www.slate.com/articles/news_and_politics/fighting_

words/2008/08/the_verbal_revolution.html. Accessed May 20, 2018.

6. Auden WH. *Lullaby.* Academy of American Poets Website. From *Another Time,* by WH Auden. Random House; 1940. https://www. poets.org/poetsorg/poem/lullaby-0. Accessed May 20, 2018.

7. Truth Commission: South Africa. United States Institute of Peace Website. https://www.usip.org/publications/1995/12/ truth-commission-south-africa. Accessed May 20, 2018.

8. Fortin J. The Statue at the Center of Charlottesville's Storm. *The New York Times.* August 13, 2017. https://www.nytimes.com/2017/ 08/13/us/charlottesville-rally-protest-statue.html?mcubz=1. Accessed May 20, 2018.

9. The New York Times. How the Violence Unfolded in Charlottesville. Online video clip. YouTube Website. https://www.youtube.com/ watch?v=dSS1G1MP6Cs. Accessed May 20, 2018.

10. Spencer H, Dickerson C. Heather Heyer, Charlottesville Victim, Cannot Be Silenced, Mother Says. *The New York Times.* August 16, 2017. https://www.nytimes.com/2017/08/16/us/charlottesville-heather-heyer-memorial-mother.html. Accessed May 20, 2018.

11. Merica D. Trump Condemns "Hatred, Bigotry and Violence on Many Sides" in Charlottesville. *CNNPolitics.* August 13, 2017. https://www.cnn.com/2017/08/12/politics/trump-statement-alt-right-protests/index.html. Accessed May 20, 2018.

12. Trauma. American Psychological Association Website. http:// www.apa.org/topics/trauma/. Accessed May 20, 2018.

13. Key Injury and Violence Data. Centers for Disease Control and Prevention Website. https://www.cdc.gov/injury/wisqars/ overview/key_data.html. Updated May 8, 2017. Accessed May 20, 2018.

14. Depression, Trauma, and PTSD. US Department of Veterans Affairs Website. https://www.ptsd.va.gov/public/problems/depression-and-trauma.asp. Updated August 13, 2015. Accessed May 20, 2018.

15. Brady KT, Back SE. Childhood trauma, posttraumatic stress disorder, and alcohol dependence. *Alcohol Research: Current Reviews.* 2012;34(4):408–13.

16. Barnes LL, Mendes de Leon CF, Lewis TT, Bienias JL, Wilson RS, Evans DA. Perceived discrimination and mortality in a population-based study of older adults. *American Journal of Public Health.* 2008;98(7):1241–47.

17. Neiwert D. When White Nationalists Chant Their Weird Slogans, What Do They Mean? Southern Poverty Law Center Website. https://www.splcenter.org/hatewatch/2017/10/10/when-white-nationalists-chant-their-weird-slogans-what-do-they-mean.Published October 10, 2017. Accessed May 20, 2018.

18. Green E. Why the Charlottesville Marchers Were Obsessed with Jews. *The Atlantic.* August 15, 2017. https://www.theatlantic.com/politics/archive/2017/08/nazis-racism-charlottesville/536928/. Accessed May 20, 2018.

19. Washington Post staff. Deconstructing the Symbols and Slogans Spotted in Charlottesville. *The Washington Post.* August 18, 2017. https://www.washingtonpost.com/graphics/2017/local/charlottesville-videos/?utm_term=.44265344ff3e. Accessed May 20, 2018.

20. CNN. Does Donald Trump Think Muslims Are a Problem (CNN interview with Don Lemon). Online video clip. YouTube Website. https://www.youtube.com/watch?v=RoLjObigUNA. Accessed May 20, 2018.

21. Lopez G. We Need to Stop Acting Like Trump Isn't Pandering to White Supremacists. *Vox.* August 14, 2017. https://www. vox.com/policy-and-politics/2017/8/13/16140504/trump-charlottesville-white-supremacists. Accessed May 20, 2018.

22. Dawsey J. Trump Derides Protections for Immigrants from "Shithole" Countries. *The Washington Post.* January 12, 2018. https:// www.washingtonpost.com/politics/trump-attacks-protections-for-immigrants-from-shithole-countries-in-oval-office-meeting/ 2018/01/11/bfc0725c-f711-11e7-91af-31ac729add94_story. html?utm_term=.aabb097282fa. Accessed May 20, 2018.

23. Jefferson T, et al. The Declaration of Independence. USHistory. org Website. http://www.ushistory.org/declaration/document/ . Accessed May 20, 2018.

24. Applestein D. The Three-Fifths Compromise: Rationalizing the Irrational. National Constitution Center Website. https:// constitutioncenter.org/blog/the-three-fifths-compromise-rationalizing-the-irrational/. Published February 12, 2013. Accessed May 20, 2018.

25. Lithwick D, Stern MJ. Consequences in Texas. *Slate.* August 25, 2017. http://www.slate.com/articles/news_and_politics/juris-prudence/2017/08/an_era_of_racist_voter_id_laws_in_texas_may_be_coming_to_an_end.html. Accessed May 20, 2018.

26. Haake G, Franco A, Clark D, Rosenberg J. Thousands March in Boston for Counter-Protest to "Free Speech Rally." *NBC News.* August 19, 2017. https://www.nbcnews.com/news/us-news/ thousands-march-boston-counter-protest-free-speech-rally-n794156. Accessed May 20, 2018.

27. Gambino L, Siddiqui S, Owen P, Helmore E. Thousands Protest Against Trump Travel Ban in Cities and Airports Nationwide. *The Guardian.* January 29, 2017. https://www.theguardian.com/

us-news/2017/jan/29/protest-trump-travel-ban-muslims-airports. Accessed May 20, 2018.

28. Moseley A. Philosophy of Love. Internet Encyclopedia of Philosophy Website. http://www.iep.utm.edu/love/#SH1c. Accessed May 20, 2018.

29. Popova M. An Experiment in Love: Martin Luther King, Jr. on the Six Pillars of Nonviolent Resistance and the Ancient Greek Notion of "Agape." *Brain Pickings.* https://www.brainpickings.org/2015/07/01/martin-luther-king-jr-an-experiment-in-love/. Accessed May 20, 2018.

30. The Holy Bible: King James Version. MLibrary Digital Collections – University of Michigan. https://quod.lib.umich.edu/cgi/k/kjv/kjv-idx?type=citation&book=Matthew&chapn o=22&startverse=34&endverse=40. Accessed May 20, 2018.

31. Galea S, Tracy M, Hoggatt KJ, DiMaggio C, Karpati A. Estimated deaths attributable to social factors in the United States. *American Journal of Public Health.* 2011;101(8):1456–65.

32. Augustine. Graves D, ed. #110: Augustine's Love Sermon. Christian History Institute Website. https://christianhistoryinstitute.org/study/module/augustine. Accessed May 20, 2018.

33. Auden WH. *As I Walked Out One Evening.* Academy of American Poets Website. From *Another Time*, by WH Auden. Random House; 1940. https://www.poets.org/poetsorg/poem/i-walked-out-one-evening. Accessed May 20, 2018.

CHAPTER 8

1. Compassion. Dictionary by Merriam-Webster Website. https://www.merriam-webster.com/dictionary/compassion. Accessed May 21, 2018.

2. King, Jr. ML. "Beyond Vietnam: A Time to Break Silence." Speech delivered on April 4, 1967. American Rhetoric Website. http://www.americanrhetoric.com/speeches/mlkatimetobreaksilence.htm. Accessed May 21, 2018.

3. Martin N, Montagne R. Black Mothers Keep Dying After Giving Birth. Shalon Irving's Story Explains Why. *NPR*. December 7, 2017. https://www.npr.org/2017/12/07/568948782/black-mothers-keep-dying-after-giving-birth-shalon-irvings-story-explains-why. Accessed May 21, 2018.

4. Schopenhauer A, trans. by EFJ Payne. *On the Basis of Morality*. Providence, RI: Berghahn Books; 1995.

5. Galea S. A Public Health Lesson from Hurricane Harvey: Invest in Prevention. *Harvard Business Review*. September 1, 2017. https://hbr.org/2017/09/a-public-health-lesson-from-hurricane-harvey-invest-in-prevention. Accessed May 21, 2018.

6. Resnick B, Barclay E. What Every American Needs to Know About Puerto Rico's Hurricane Disaster. *Vox*. October 16, 2017. https://www.vox.com/science-and-health/2017/9/26/16365994/hurricane-maria-2017-puerto-rico-san-juan-humanitarian-disaster-electricty-fuel-flights-facts. Accessed May 21, 2018.

7. Levenson E. These Are the Victims of the Florida School Shooting. *CNN*. February 21, 2018. https://www.cnn.com/2018/02/15/us/florida-shooting-victims-school/index.html. Accessed May 21, 2018.

8. Galea S. The Case for Public Health, in 18 Charts. *HuffPost*. August 25, 2016. https://www.huffingtonpost.com/sandro-galea/the-case-for-public-healt_b_11699182.html. Accessed May 21, 2018.

CHAPTER 9

1. Humoral doctrine. The Free Dictionary Website. https://medical-dictionary.thefreedictionary.com/humoral+theory. Accessed May 21, 2018.

2. Iyengar S. *Shakespeare's Medical Language: A Dictionary*. Arden Shakespeare Dictionaries. New York: Bloomsbury; 2014.

3. Greenstone G. The history of bloodletting. *British Columbia Medical Journal*. 2010;52(1):12–14.

4. Epistemology. AskDefine Website. http://epistemology.askdefinebeta.com/. Accessed May 21, 2018.

5. Galea S, Ettman C, DelGizzo E. On Knowledge and Values. Boston University School of Public Health Website. https://www.bu.edu/sph/2016/10/16/on-knowledge-and-values/. Published October 16, 2016. Accessed May 21, 2018.

6. Aristotle. *Metaphysics*. Classical Wisdom Weekly Website. https://classicalwisdom.com/greek_books/metaphysics-by-aristotle-book-iv/7/. Accessed May 21, 2018.

7. Epistemology. The Basics of Philosophy Website. https://www.philosophybasics.com/branch_epistemology.html. Accessed May 21, 2018.

8. Chappell SG. Plato on Knowledge in the *Theaetetus*. Stanford Encyclopedia of Philosophy Website. https://plato.stanford.edu/entries/plato-theaetetus/. Published May 7, 2005. Updated December 13, 2013. Accessed May 21, 2018.

9. Steps of the Scientific Method. Science Buddies Website. https://www.sciencebuddies.org/science-fair-projects/science-fair/steps-of-the-scientific-method. Accessed May 21, 2018.

10. Shwed U, Bearman PS. The temporal structure of scientific consensus formation. *American Sociological Review*. 2010;75(6):817–40.

11. Galea S, DelGizzo E. How Do We Know When We Know Something? Boston University School of Public Health Website. https://www.bu.edu/sph/2017/11/05/how-do-we-know-when-we-know-something/. Published November 5, 2017. Accessed May 21, 2018.

12. Trinquart L, Johns DM, Galea S. Why do we think we know what we know? A metaknowledge analysis of the salt controversy. *International Journal of Epidemiology.* 2016;45(1):251–60.

13. Bernoulli's Principle. Encylopedia.com Website. https://www.encyclopedia.com/science-and-technology/physics/physics/bernoullis-principle. Accessed May 21, 2018.

14. Latour B. *Science in Action. How to Follow Scientists and Engineers Through Society.* Cambridge, MA: Harvard University Press; 1987.

15. Galea S. On the production of useful knowledge. *Milbank Quarterly.* 2017;95(4):722–25.

16. Galea S. On creating a national health conversation. *Milbank Quarterly.* 2018;96(1):5–8.

17. Trends in Current Cigarette Smoking Among High School Students and Adults, United States, 1965–2014. Centers for Disease Control and Prevention Website. https://www.cdc.gov/tobacco/data_statistics/tables/trends/cig_smoking/index.htm. Updated March 30, 2016. Accessed May 21, 2018.

18. Centers for Disease Control and Prevention. Achievements in public health, 1900–1999: Tobacco use. *Morbidity and Mortality Weekly Report (MMWR).* 1999;48(43):986–93.

19. Office on Smoking and Health, National Center for Chronic Disease Prevention and Health Promotion, Centers for Disease Control and Prevention. History of the Surgeon General's Reports on Smoking and Health. Centers for Disease Control and Prevention Website. https://www.cdc.gov/tobacco/data_statistics/sgr/history/index.htm. Updated July 6, 2009. Accessed May 21, 2018.

20. Health Impact in 5 Years. Centers for Disease Control and Prevention Website. https://www.cdc.gov/policy/hst/hi5/index.html. Updated October 21, 2016. Accessed May 21, 2018.

21. Glynn I, Glynn J. *The Life and Death of Smallpox*. Cambridge: Cambridge University Press; 2004.

22. Public Health Historian, History of Medicine Division, National Library of Medicine, National Institutes of Health. Smallpox: A Great and Terrible Scourge. US National Library of Medicine Website. https://www.nlm.nih.gov/exhibition/smallpox/sp_resistance.html. Published October 18, 2002. Updated July 30, 2013. Accessed May 21, 2018.

23. Inoculation. Thomas Jefferson's Monticello Website. https://www.monticello.org/site/research-and-collections/inoculation Accessed September 7, 2018.

24. UN Agencies, Partners to Launch Polio Vaccination Campaign Across Africa. *UN News*. March 24, 2017. https://news.un.org/en/story/2017/03/553932-un-agencies-partners-launch-polio-vaccination-campaign-across-africa. Accessed May 21, 2018.

25. Disease Eradication. History of Vaccines Website. https://www.historyofvaccines.org/content/articles/disease-eradication. Updated January 25, 2018. Accessed May 21, 2018.

26. 10 Facts on Polio Eradication. World Health Organization Website. http://www.who.int/features/factfiles/polio/en/. Updated April 2017. Accessed May 21, 2018.

CHAPTER 10

1. Epstein J. *Fred Astaire*. New Haven, CT: Yale University Press; 2008.

2. Sara Smith I. Fred Astaire (1899–1987). Dance Heritage Coalition Website. http://www.danceheritage.org/treasures/astaire_essay_smith2.pdf. Accessed May 21, 2018.

3. Giles S. *Fred Astaire: His Friends Talk.* New York: Doubleday; 1988.

4. Lerner AJ. *The Street Where I Live.* New York: Norton; 1978.

5. Novey B. Can We Finally Stop Doing Things "Backwards and in Heels"? *NPR.* August 4, 2016. https://www.npr.org/sections/monkeysee/2016/08/04/488213995/can-we-finally-stop-doing-things-backwards-and-in-heels. Accessed May 21, 2018.

6. Hanson RT. Dancin' Fools: The Art of Fred Astaire and Gene Kelly. Humanities Seminar Program—University of Arizona Website. https://hsp.arizona.edu/course/dancin-fools-art-fred-astaire-and-gene-kelly. Accessed May 21, 2018.

7. Jones J. Master of Style, Elegance Was 88: Fred Astaire, Movies' Greatest Dancer, Dies. *Los Angeles Times.* June 23, 1987. http://articles.latimes.com/1987-06-23/news/mn-10167_1_fred-astaire. Accessed May 21, 2018.

8. Knopper S. Inside Michael Jackson's Iconic First Moonwalk Onstage. *Rolling Stone.* October 5, 2015. https://www.rollingstone.com/music/news/inside-michael-jackson-s-iconic-first-moonwalk-onstage-20151005. Accessed May 21, 2018.

9. Green A. How Jackie Chan Draws Inspiration from Classic Hollywood. *Mental Floss.* February 16, 2016. http://mentalfloss.com/article/75546/how-jackie-chan-draws-inspiration-classic-hollywood. Accessed May 21, 2018.

10. Wills G. *Certain Trumpets: The Call of Leaders.* New York: Simon & Schuster; 1994.

11. The Public Health Impact of Chemicals: Knowns and Unknowns. World Health Organization Website. http://www.who.int/ipcs/publications/chemicals-public-health-impact/en/ Accessed September 7, 2018.

12. Galea S, Riddle M, Kaplan GA. Causal thinking and complex system approaches in epidemiology. *International Journal of Epidemiology.* 2010;39(1):97–106.

13. Wright JC, Nadelhoffer T, Perini T, Langville A, Echols M, Venezia K. The psychological significance of humility. *The Journal of Positive Psychology.* 2017;12(1):3–12.

14. Sokol DK. "First do no harm" revisited. *The BMJ.* 2013;347: f6426.

15. Mukherjee S. New Zealand Is About to Make the Revolutionary HIV Prevention Drug Truvada Almost Free. *Fortune.* February 7, 2018. http://fortune.com/2018/02/07/new-zealand-hiv-prep-truvada/. Accessed May 22, 2018.

16. HIV and AIDS in South Africa. Avert Website. https://www.avert.org/professionals/hiv-around-world/sub-saharan-africa/south-africa. Accessed May 22, 2018.

17. Halliday S. Death and miasma in Victorian London: an obstinate belief. *The BMJ.* 2001;323(7327):1469–71.

18. Cholera. WebMD Website. https://www.webmd.com/a-to-z-guides/cholera-faq#1. Accessed May 22, 2018.

19. Tuthill K, illustrated by Van Wyk R. John Snow and the Broad Street Pump: on the trail of an epidemic. *Cricket.* 2003;31(3):23–31.

20. Black A. Broad Street Cholera Pump. Atlas Obscura Website. https://www.atlasobscura.com/places/broad-street-cholera-pump. Accessed May 22, 2018.

21. Marlowe C. *The Tragical History of Doctor Faustus,* ed. by The Rev. Alexander Dyce. Project Gutenberg Website. https://www.gutenberg.org/files/779/779-h/779-h.htm. Accessed May 22, 2018.

22. Stevenson RL. *The Strange Case of Dr. Jekyll and Mr. Hyde.* Project Gutenberg Website. https://www.gutenberg.org/files/43/43-h/43-h.htm. Accessed May 22, 2018.

23. Shelley M. *Frankenstein; or, the Modern Prometheus.* Project Gutenberg Website. https://www.gutenberg.org/files/84/84-h/84-h.htm. Accessed May 22, 2018.

24. Galea S, Tracy M, Hoggatt KJ, Dimaggio C, Karpati A. Estimated deaths attributable to social factors in the United States. *American Journal of Public Health.* 2011;101(8):1456–65.

CHAPTER 11

1. Fulbright JW. The American experiment in self-government. *The Virginia Magazine of History and Biography.* 1955;63(2):151–60.

2. Coates T. What This Cruel War Was Over. *The Atlantic.* June 22, 2015. https://www.theatlantic.com/politics/archive/2015/06/what-this-cruel-war-was-over/396482/. Accessed May 22, 2018.

3. *United Daughters of the Confederacy Magazine.* 1957. From Confederate Past Present Website. http://www.confederatepastpresent.org/index.php?option=com_content&view=article&id=88:confederate-princples-yesterday-and-today-oct-nov-1957&catid=36:the-civil-rights-era&Itemid=47. Accessed March 15, 2018.

4. *Brown v. Board of Education.* History Website. https://www.history.com/topics/black-history/brown-v-board-of-education-of-topeka. Accessed May 23, 2018.

5. Valant J. Donald Trump, Betsy DeVos, and the Changing Politics of Charter Schools. Brookings Website. https://www.brookings.edu/blog/brown-center-chalkboard/2017/02/07/donald-trump-betsy-devos-and-the-changing-politics-of-charter-schools/. Published February 7, 2017. Accessed May 23, 2018.

6. Moffit R. Obamacare and the Individual Mandate: Violating Personal Liberty and Federalism. The Heritage Foundation Website. https://www.heritage.org/health-care-reform/report/obamacare-and-the-individual-mandate-violating-personal-liberty-and.Published January 18, 2011. Accessed May 23, 2018.

7. Bandow D. Gun Rights and Liberty Go Hand in Hand. Cato Institute Website (originally appeared in *Investor's Business Daily*). https://www.cato.org/publications/commentary/gun-rights-liberty-go-hand-hand. Accessed May 23, 2018.

8. Reagan R. "Inaugural Address." January 20, 1981. Online by Gerhard Peters and John T. Woolley. The American Presidency Project Website. http://www.presidency.ucsb.edu/ws/?pid=43130. Accessed May 23, 2018.

9. Galea S. Why The Trump Administration Is Hazardous to Your Health. *Cognoscenti*. March 12, 2018. http://www.wbur.org/cognoscenti/2018/03/12/trump-health-life-expectancy-sandro-galea. Accessed May 23, 2018.

10. Lindsey R. A Cowboy Hero, Myth and Reality. *The New York Times*. 1981. https://www.nytimes.com/1981/01/21/us/a-cowboy-hero-myth-and-reality.html. Accessed May 23, 2018.

11. Homestead Act. History Website. https://www.history.com/topics/homestead-act. Accessed May 23, 2018.

12. Homestead Act (1862). Our Documents Website. https://www.ourdocuments.gov/doc.php?flash=true&doc=31. Accessed May 23, 2018.

13. The Homestead Act of 1862. National Archives Website. https://www.archives.gov/education/lessons/homestead-act. Accessed May 23, 2018.

14. The Last Homesteader. National Park Service Website. https://www.nps.gov/home/learn/historyculture/lasthomesteader.htm. Accessed May 23, 2018.

15. Roosevelt FD. "State of the Union Message to Congress." January 11, 1944. Franklin D. Roosevelt Presidential Library and Museum Website. http://www.fdrlibrary.marist.edu/archives/address_text.html. Accessed May 23, 2018.

16. Bradley A. Positive rights, negative rights and health care. *Journal of Medical Ethics.* 2010;36(12):838–41.

CHAPTER 12

1. *The Devil Wears Prada* (film). Directed by David Frankel. USA: 20th Century Fox; 2006.

2. Overweight & Obesity Statistics. National Institute of Diabetes and Digestive and Kidney Diseases Website. https://www.niddk.nih.gov/health-information/health-statistics/overweight-obesity. Accessed May 22, 2018.

3. The Healthcare Costs of Obesity. The State of Obesity Website. https://stateofobesity.org/healthcare-costs-obesity/. Accessed May 22, 2018.

4. Galea S, DelGizzo E. Meeting the Challenge of Obesity. Boston University School of Public Health Website. https://www.bu.edu/sph/2016/10/09/meeting-the-challenge-of-obesity/. Accessed May 22, 2018.

5. Larger Portion Sizes Contribute to US Obesity Problem. National Heart, Lung, and Blood Institute Website. https://www.nhlbi.nih.gov/health/educational/wecan/news-events/matte1.htm. Updated February 13, 2013. Accessed May 22, 2018.

6. Shen A. The Disastrous Legacy of Nancy Reagan's "Just Say No" Campaign. *ThinkProgress.* March 6, 2016. https://thinkprogress.org/the-disastrous-legacy-of-nancy-reagans-just-say-no-campaign-fd24570bf109/. Accessed May 22, 2018.

7. The Science of Drug Abuse and Addiction: The Basics. National Institute on Drug Abuse Website. https://www.drugabuse.gov/

publications/media-guide/science-drug-abuse-addiction-basics. Accessed May 22, 2018.

8. Sullivan A. The Poison We Pick. *New York* Magazine. February 20, 2018. http://nymag.com/daily/intelligencer/2018/02/americas-opioid-epidemic.html. Accessed May 20, 2018.

9. Lopez G. The Maker of OxyContin Will Finally Stop Marketing the Addictive Opioid to Doctors. *Vox.* February 12, 2018. https://www.vox.com/science-and-health/2018/2/12/16998122/opioid-crisis-oxycontin-purdue-advertising. Accessed May 20, 2018.

10. Florida R. The Real Cause of the Opioid Crisis. *CityLab.* February 14, 2018. https://www.citylab.com/life/2018/02/the-real-cause-of-the-opioid-crisis/553118/. Accessed May 20, 2018.

11. Hornik R, Jacobsohn L, Orwin R, Piesse A, Kalton G. Effects of the national youth anti-drug media campaign on youths. *American Journal of Public Health.* 2008;98(12):2229–36.

12. Young NJ. The NRA Wasn't Always a Front for Gun Makers. *HuffPost.* February 24, 2018. https://www.huffingtonpost.com/entry/opinion-young-nra-history_us_5a907fbee4b03b55731c2169. Accessed May 20, 2018.

13. The DDT Story. Pesticide Action Network Website. http://www.panna.org/resources/ddt-story. Accessed May 20, 2018.

14. Paltzer S. The Other Foe: The US Army's Fight Against Malaria in the Pacific Theater, 1942–45. Army Historical Foundation Website. https://armyhistory.org/the-other-foe-the-u-s-armys-fight-against-malaria-in-the-pacific-theater-1942-45/. Accessed May 20, 2018.

15. American Chemical Society National Historic Chemical Landmarks. Rachel Carson's *Silent Spring.* American Chemical Society Website. https://www.acs.org/content/acs/en/education/whatischemistry/landmarks/rachel-carson-silent-spring.html. Accessed May 20, 2018.

16. The Story of Silent Spring. Natural Resources Defense Council Website. https://www.nrdc.org/stories/story-silent-spring. Published August 13, 2015. Accessed May 20, 2018.

17. Conis E. Beyond Silent Spring: An Alternate History of DDT. *Distillations*. Winter 2017. https://www.sciencehistory.org/distillations/magazine/beyond-silent-spring-an-alternate-history-of-ddt. Accessed May 20, 2018.

18. Lewis J. The Birth of EPA. US Environmental Protection Agency Website. https://archive.epa.gov/epa/aboutepa/birth-epa.html. Accessed May 20, 2018.

19. Bader P, Boisclair D, Ferrence R. Effects of tobacco taxation and pricing on smoking behavior in high risk populations: a knowledge synthesis. *International Journal of Environmental Research and Public Health*. 2011;8(11):4118–39.

20. Brownell KD, Frieden TR. Ounces of prevention: the public policy case for taxes on sugared beverages. *The New England Journal of Medicine*. 2009;360(18):1805–08.

21. Weiner R. The New York City Soda Ban Explained. *The Washington Post*. March 11, 2013. https://www.washingtonpost.com/news/the-fix/wp/2013/03/11/the-new-york-city-soda-ban-explained/?utm_term=.e2d1b6eaf06f. Accessed May 20, 2018.

22. Grynbaum MM. New York's Ban on Big Sodas Is Rejected by Final Court. *The New York Times*. June 26, 2014. https://www.nytimes.com/2014/06/27/nyregion/city-loses-final-appeal-on-limiting-sales-of-large-sodas.html. Accessed May 20, 2018.

23. Galoozis C. A New Kind of Paternalism. *Harvard Political Review*. October 27, 2012. http://harvardpolitics.com/united-states/a-new-kind-of-paternalism/. Accessed May 20, 2018.

CHAPTER 13

1. Fortuna. Encyclopedia Britannica Website. https://www. britannica.com/topic/Fortuna-Roman-goddess. Accessed May 22, 2018.

2. Tomasetti C, Li L, Vogelstein B. Stem cell divisions, somatic mutations, cancer etiology, and cancer prevention. *Science.* 2017;355(6331):1330–34.

3. Harris R. Cancer Is Partly Caused by Bad Luck, Study Finds. *NPR.* March 23, 2017. https://www.npr.org/sections/health-shots/2017/03/23/521219318/cancer-is-partly-caused-by-bad-luck-study-finds. Accessed May 22, 2018.

4. Cassidy J. Piketty's Inequality Story in Six Charts. *The New Yorker.* March 26, 2014. https://www.newyorker.com/news/john-cassidy/pikettys-inequality-story-in-six-charts. Accessed May 22, 2018.

5. Mason A. Equality of Opportunity. Encyclopedia Britannica Websitlooe. https://www.britannica.com/topic/equality-of-opportunity#ref1187627. Accessed May 22, 2018.

6. Chait J. Republican Blurts Out That Sick People Don't Deserve Affordable Care. *New York* Magazine. May 1, 2017. http://nymag. com/daily/intelligencer/2017/05/republican-sick-people-dont-deserve-affordable-care.html. Accessed May 22, 2018.

7. Gun Violence by the Numbers. Everytown for Gun Safety Website. https://everytownresearch.org/gun-violence-by-the-numbers/#BlackAmericans. Accessed May 22, 2018.

CHAPTER 14

1. *Star Trek II: The Wrath of Khan* (film). Directed by Nicholas Meyer. USA: Paramount Pictures; 1982.

2. Gene Roddenberry. America and the Utopian Dream: Yale University Website. http://brbl-archive.library.yale.edu/exhibitions/utopia/ut15.html. Accessed May 22, 2018.

3. Burns JH. Happiness and utility: Jeremy Bentham's equation. *Utilitas*. 2005;17(1):46–61.

4. Katz J. The First Count of Fentanyl Deaths in 2016: Up 540% in Three Years. *The New York Times*. September 2, 2017. https://www.nytimes.com/interactive/2017/09/02/upshot/fentanyl-drug-overdose-deaths.html. Accessed May 22, 2018.

5. Slovic P, Finucane ML, Peters E, MacGregor DG. Risk as analysis and risk as feelings: some thoughts about affect, reason, risk, and rationality. *Risk Analysis*. 2004;24(2):311–22.

6. Galea S. Obamacare Is Not Enough. *US News & World Report*. June 15, 2016. https://www.usnews.com/opinion/articles/2016-06-15/obamacare-is-not-enough-to-improve-americans-health. Accessed May 22, 2018.

7. Fletcher H. Q&A: Dr. Tony Iton: "What's in the Way of the American Dream Right Now?" *BirdDog*. March 21, 2018. https://readbirddog.com/2018/03/21/dr-tony-iton-on-why-american-dream-is-faltering/. Accessed May 22, 2018.

8. Life Expectancy at Birth (Years), 2000–2016: Both Sexes: 2016. Life expectancy. WHO Website. http://gamapserver.who.int/gho/interactive_charts/mbd/life_expectancy/atlas.html. Accessed May 22, 2018.

9. Molina RL, Pace LE. A renewed focus on maternal health in the United States. *The New England Journal of Medicine*. 2017;377(18):1705–07.

10. Impaired Driving: Get the Facts. Centers for Disease Control and Prevention Website. https://www.cdc.gov/motorvehiclesafety/

impaired_driving/impaired-drv_factsheet.html. Updated June 16, 2017. Accessed May 22, 2018.

11. Community Water Fluoridation. Centers for Disease Control and Prevention Website. https://www.cdc.gov/fluorida-tion/index.html. Updated February 21, 2018. Accessed May 22, 2018.

12. Mind-Meld, Vulcan. Star Trek Website. http://www.startrek.com/database_article/mind-meld-vulcan. Accessed May 22, 2018.

13. Star Trek: The Original Series. Memory Alpha Website. http://memory-alpha.wikia.com/wiki/Star_Trek:_The_Original_Series. Accessed May 22, 2018.

CHAPTER 15

1. Dickens C. *A Christmas Carol in Prose, Being a Ghost-Story of Christmas.* Project Gutenberg Website. http://www.gutenberg.org/files/46/46-h/46-h.htm. Accessed May 23, 2018.

2. Effects of the Industrial Revolution. Modern World History Website. https://webs.bcp.org/sites/vcleary/modernworldhistorytextbook/industrialrevolution/ireffects.html#Urbanization. Accessed May 23, 2018.

3. Editorial. The New Resentment of the Poor. *The New York Times.* August 30, 2011. https://www.nytimes.com/2011/08/31/opinion/the-new-resentment-of-the-poor.html?_r=1&hp. Accessed May 23, 2018.

4. Colgrove J. The McKeown thesis: a historical controversy and its enduring influence. *American Journal of Public Health.* 2002;92(5):725–29.

5. How Has Life Expectancy Changed over Time? Office for National Statistics Website. https://www.ons.gov.uk/peoplepopulationandcommunity/birthsdeathsandmarriages/lifeexpectancies/articles/howhaslifeexpectancychangedovertime/2015-09-09. Published September 9, 2015. Accessed May 23, 2018.

6. Pappas S. Dickensian Diagnosis: Tiny Tim's Symptoms Decoded. Live Science Website. https://www.livescience.com/18802-dickens-tiny-tim-diagnosis.html. Published March 5, 2012. Accessed May 23, 2018.

7. Bowyer J. What Was Charles Dickens Really Doing When He Wrote "A Christmas Carol"? *Forbes*. December 11, 2013. https://www.forbes.com/sites/jerrybowyer/2013/12/11/what-was-charles-dickens-really-doing-when-he-wrote-a-christmas-carol/#57e9a23b7db8. Accessed May 23, 2018.

8. Weller C. These Charts Show the World Is Better Than Ever—Even If Things Seem Apocalyptic. *Business Insider*. September 18, 2017. http://www.businessinsider.com/charts-global-progress-humanity-getting-better-2017-9. Accessed May 23, 2018.

9. Case A, Deaton A. Rising morbidity and mortality in mid-life among white non-Hispanic Americans in the 21st century. *Proceedings of the National Academy of Sciences of the United States of America*. 2015;112(49):15078–83.

10. Vance JD. *Hillbilly Elegy*. New York: Harper; 2016.

11. Average Number of People per Household in the United States from 1960 to 2017. Statista Website. https://www.statista.com/statistics/183648/average-size-of-households-in-the-us/. Accessed May 23, 2018.

12. Vo LT. What Americans Earn. *NPR*. July 16, 2012. https://www.npr.org/sections/money/2012/07/16/156688596/what-americans-earn. Accessed May 23, 2018.

13. Bor J, Cohen GH, Galea S. Population health in an era of rising income inequality: USA, 1980–2015. *The Lancet*. 2017;389(10077):1475–90.

14. Wolff EN. Household Wealth Trends in the United States, 1962 to 2016: Has Middle Class Wealth Recovered? Working paper. The National Bureau of Economic Research Website. http://www.nber.org/papers/w24085.pdf. Accessed May 23, 2018.

15. Scapegoat. Dictionary.com Website. http://www.dictionary.com/browse/scapegoat. Accessed May 23, 2018.

16. What Climate Change Means for Africa, Asia and the Coastal Poor. World Bank Website. http://www.worldbank.org/en/news/feature/2013/06/19/what-climate-change-means-africa-asia-coastal-poor. Published June 19, 2013. Accessed May 23, 2018.

17. Dewan TH. Societal impacts and vulnerability to floods in Bangladesh and Nepal. *Weather and Climate Extremes*. 2015;7:36–42.

18. Shultz JM, et al. Risks, health consequences, and response challenges for small-island-based populations: observations from the 2017 Atlantic hurricane season. *Disaster Medicine and Public Health Preparedness*. 2018:1–13.

19. Galea S, Annas GJ. Aspirations and strategies for public health. *JAMA: The Journal of the American Medical Association*. 2016;315(7):655–56.

CHAPTER 16

1. Public Good. Investopedia Website. https://www.investopedia.com/terms/p/public-good.asp. Accessed May 23, 2018.

2. Private Good. Investopedia Website. https://www.investopedia.com/terms/p/private-good.asp. Accessed May 23, 2018.

3. Martin D, Galea S. O Canada: What Our Neighbors to the North Can Teach Us About Health Care Reform. *STAT*. March 27, 2017. https://www.statnews.com/2017/03/27/health-care-reform-canada-us/. Accessed May 23, 2018.

CHAPTER 17

1. Kwiff Official. Random Act of Unfairness. Online video clip. YouTube Website. https://www.youtube.com/watch?v=_lT4JqfOGKk. Accessed May 24, 2018.

2. Fairness. Cambridge Dictionary Website. https://dictionary.cambridge.org/us/dictionary/english/fairness. Accessed May 24, 2018.

3. Graf N, Brown A, Patten E. The Narrowing, but Persistent, Gender Gap in Pay. Pew Research Center Website. http://www.pewresearch.org/fact-tank/2018/04/09/gender-pay-gap-facts/. Published April 9, 2018. Accessed May 24, 2018.

4. Benz JK, Espinosa O, Welsh V, Fontes A. Awareness of racial and ethnic health disparities has improved only modestly over a decade. *Health Affairs*. 2011;30(10):1860–67.

5. Black Americans and HIV/AIDS: The Basics. Kaiser Family Foundation Website. https://www.kff.org/hivaids/fact-sheet/black-americans-and-hivaids-the-basics/. Published February 6, 2018. Accessed May 24, 2018.

6. Latinos and HIV/AIDS. Kaiser Family Foundation Website. https://www.kff.org/hivaids/fact-sheet/latinos-and-hivaids/. Published April 15, 2014. Accessed May 24, 2018.

7. Martin M, Foner E. Interview. End of Slave Trade Meant New Normal for America. *NPR*. January 10, 2008. https://www.npr.org/templates/story/story.php?storyId=17988106. Accessed May 24, 2018.

8. Hunter TW. Putting an Antebellum Myth to Rest. *The New York Times*. August 1, 2011. https://www.nytimes.com/2011/08/02/opinion/putting-an-antebellum-myth-about-slave-families-to-rest.html. Accessed May 24, 2018.

9. Treatment. Thomas Jefferson's Monticello Website. https://www.monticello.org/mulberry-row/topics/treatment. Accessed May 24, 2018.

10. Thomas Jefferson's Attitudes Toward Slavery. Thomas Jefferson's Monticello Website. https://www.monticello.org/site/plantation-and-slavery/thomas-jeffersons-attitudes-toward-slavery. Accessed May 24, 2018.

CHAPTER 18

1. Jones JM. US Concerns About Healthcare High; Energy, Unemployment Low. Gallup Website. http://news.gallup.com/poll/231533/concerns-healthcare-high-energy-unemployment-low.aspx?utm_source=alert&utm_medium=email&utm_content=morelink&utm_campaign=syndication. Published March 26, 2018. Accessed May 24, 2018.

2. Griffin S, Cubanski J, Neuman T, Jankiewicz A, Rousseau D; Kaiser Family Foundation. Medicare and end-of-life care. *JAMA: The Journal of the American Medical Association*. 2016;316(17):1754.

3. Dieleman JL, et al. Factors associated with increases in US health care spending, 1996–2013. *JAMA: The Journal of the American Medical Association*. 2017;318(17):1668–78.

4. Annas GJ, Galea S. Dying Healthy: Public Health Priorities for Fixed Population Life Expectancies. *Annals of Internal Medicine*. 2018;168(8).

5. How to Live Longer Better, February 26, 2018 issue. TIME Website. http://time.com/magazine/us/5159845/february-26th-2018-vol-191-no-7-u-s/. Accessed May 24, 2018.

6. Dong X, Milholland B, Vijg J. Evidence for a limit to human lifespan. *Nature.* 2016;538:257–59.

7. Constitution of WHO: Principles. World Health Organization Website. http://www.who.int/about/mission/en/. Accessed May 24, 2018.

8. O'Keefe T. Epicurus (341–271 BCE). Internet Encyclopedia of Philosophy Website. http://www.iep.utm.edu/epicur/#SH5b. Accessed May 24, 2018.

9. Duignan B, Diano C. Epicureanism. Encyclopedia Britannica Website. https://www.britannica.com/topic/Epicureanism. Accessed May 24, 2018.

10. Hedonism. Encyclopedia Britannica Website. https://www.britannica.com/topic/hedonism. Updated April 6, 2018. Accessed May 24, 2018.

11. Bentham J. *An Introduction to the Principles of Morals and Legislation.* Oxford: Clarendon Press; 1907 reprint of 1823 edition.

12. Zera. Jeremy Bentham: Felicific Calculus. Economic Theories Website. http://www.economictheories.org/2008/12/jeremy-bentham-felicific-calculus.html. Accessed May 24, 2018.

13. Soares MO. Is the QALY blind, deaf and dumb to equity? NICE's considerations over equity. *British Medical Bulletin.* 2012;101:17–31.

14. Moolgavkar SH, et al. Impact of reduced tobacco smoking on lung cancer mortality in the United States during 1975–2000. *Journal of the National Cancer Institute.* 2012;104(7):541–48.

CHAPTER 19

1. Shakespeare W. *The Tragedy of Hamlet, Prince of Denmark*. The Complete Works of William Shakespeare: MIT Website. http://shakespeare.mit.edu/hamlet/index.html. Accessed May 24, 2018.

2. Bevington D. Hamlet. Encyclopedia Britannica Website. https://www.britannica.com/topic/Hamlet-by-Shakespeare. Updated March 29, 2018. Accessed May 24, 2018.

3. Shapiro J. How Shakespeare's Great Escape from the Plague Changed Theatre. *The Guardian*. September 24, 2015. https://www.theguardian.com/books/2015/sep/24/shakespeares-great-escape-plague-1606--james-shapiro. Accessed May 24, 2018.

4. Plague (*Yersinia pestis*). Drugs.com Website. https://www.drugs.com/health-guide/plague-yersinia-pestis.html. Accessed May 24, 2018.

5. Plague. Boston Public Health Commission Website. http://www.bphc.org/whatwedo/infectious-diseases/Infectious-Diseases-A-to-Z/Pages/Plague.aspx. Accessed May 24, 2018.

6. London Plagues 1348–1665. Museum of London Website. https://www.museumoflondon.org.uk/application/files/5014/5434/6066/london-plagues-1348-1665.pdf. Accessed May 24, 2018.

7. Plague: Symptoms. Centers for Disease Control and Prevention Website. https://www.cdc.gov/plague/symptoms/index.html. Updated September 14, 2015. Accessed May 24, 2018.

8. Benedictow OJ. The Black Death: The Greatest Catastrophe Ever. *History Today*. March 2005. https://www.historytoday.com/ole-j-benedictow/black-death-greatest-catastrophe-ever. Accessed May 24, 2018.

9. George P. Memento Mori—remember that you have to die. *The Conversation*. June 21, 2015. https://theconversation.com/

memento-mori-remember-that-you-have-to-die-42823. Accessed May 24, 2018.

10. Memento Mori. Tate Modern Website. http://www.tate.org.uk/art/art-terms/m/memento-mori. Accessed May 24, 2018.

11. Shakespeare W. Sonnet 60. Shakespeare Online Website. http://www.shakespeare-online.com/sonnets/60.html. Accessed May 24, 2018.

12. Favor. Merriam-Webster Website. https://www.merriam-webster.com/dictionary/favor. Accessed May 24, 2018.

13. Picard L. Cities in Elizabethan England. The British Library Website. https://www.bl.uk/shakespeare/articles/cities-in-elizabethan-england. Published March 15, 2016. Accessed May 24, 2018.

14. Briscoe A. Poverty in Elizabethan England. *BBC*. http://www.bbc.co.uk/history/british/tudors/poverty_01.shtml#five. Updated February 17, 2011. Accessed May 24, 2018.

15. Daily Life in the Elizabethan Era. Encyclopedia.com Website. https://www.encyclopedia.com/humanities/news-wires-white-papers-and-books/daily-life-elizabethan-era. Accessed May 24, 2018.

16. National Life Tables, UK: 2013–2015. Office for National Statistics Website. https://www.ons.gov.uk/peoplepopulationandcommunity/birthsdeathsandmarriages/lifeexpectancies/bulletins/nationallifetablesunitedkingdom/20132015. Accessed May 24, 2018.

17. US: Life Expectancy All Races. World Life Expectancy Website. http://www.worldlifeexpectancy.com/usa/life-expectancy. Accessed May 24, 2018.

18. Vanitas. Encyclopedia Britannica Website. https://www.britannica.com/art/vanitas-art. Accessed May 24, 2018.

19. Waldrop DP. Denying and defying death: the culture of dying in 21st century America. *The Gerontologist*. 2011;51(4):571–76.

20. Clark D. Between hope and acceptance: the medicalisation of dying. *The BMJ*. 2002;324(7342):905–7.

21. Mather M. Fact Sheet: Aging in the United States. Population Reference Bureau Website. https://www.prb.org/aging-unitedstates-fact-sheet/. Published January 13, 2016. Accessed May 24, 2018.

22. Seneca, trans. by Richard Mott Gummere. *Moral letters to Lucilius*. Aegitas; 2015.

CHAPTER 20

1. Wilkinson A, Fairhead J. Comparison of social resistance to Ebola response in Sierra Leone and Guinea suggests explanations lie in political configurations not culture. *Critical Public Health*. 2017;27(1):14–27.

2. Obesity and Cancer. National Cancer Institute Website. https://www.cancer.gov/about-cancer/causes-prevention/risk/obesity/obesity-fact-sheet#q3. Accessed May 24, 2018.

3. Adams N. The Inspiring Force of "We Shall Overcome." *NPR*. August 28, 2013. https://www.npr.org/2013/08/28/216482943/the-inspiring-force-of-we-shall-overcome. Accessed May 24, 2018.

4. Kindig J. Selma, Alabama (Bloody Sunday, March 7, 1965). The Black Past Website. http://www.blackpast.org/aah/bloody-sunday-selma-alabama-march-7-1965. Accessed May 24, 2018.

5. President Johnson's Special Message to the Congress: The American Promise. LBJ Presidential Library Website. http://www.lbjlibrary.org/lyndon-baines-johnson/speeches-films/

president-johnsons-special-message-to-the-congress-the-american-promise/. Accessed May 24, 2018.

6. Anglemyer A, Horvath T, Rutherford G. The accessibility of firearms and risk for suicide and homicide victimization among household members: a systematic review and meta-analysis. *Annals of Internal Medicine.* 2014;160(2):101–10.

7. Kristof N. How to Reduce Shootings. *The New York Times.* https://www.nytimes.com/interactive/2017/11/06/opinion/how-to-reduce-shootings.html. Updated May 18, 2018. Accessed May 24, 2018.

INDEX